Overthinking

How To Stop Worrying, Eliminate Negative Thinking, Reduce Your Anxiety and Learn Not to Give a F*ck to Live Harmoniously

By Andrew Copelan

Copyright © 2019 Andrew Copelan

All rights reserved.

Table of Contents

Introduction	7
Chapter 1: Why Are We Stressed?	16
Chapter 2: Negative Impact of Stress on Your Health, Emotions, and Psyche	22
Some of the Physical Symptoms of Stress	22
Weight Gain	28
Some of the Emotional Symptoms of Stress	30
Do Yoga	33
Chapter 3: Declutter Your Mind for Reducing Stress	39
Habits That Help You in Reducing the Mind Clutter	56
Chapter 5: Ways to Avoid Decision Fatigue	58
Choose a Role Model	61
Chapter 6: Relationships and Stress	66
Chapter 7: Understanding and Dealing with Anxiety in Dating	69
It is Very Common	70
Chapter 8: Things That Lead to Stress in Relationships	76
Chapter 9: Strategies to Improve or Eliminate Bad Relationships	83
Know Why You Want It	92
Be Patient	99
Chapter 11: 7 Steps Can Help You In Clearing Mental Clutter And Leading A Happy Life	101

Step 1: Let Go of the Baggage of the Past	101
Step 2: Eliminate Negativity from Life by Breaking Negative Thought Patterns	115
Step 3: Organize Your Mind - Control Unending Mind Chatter	130
Step 4: Curate Your Desires with Minimalism	138
Step 5: Command Ownership of Your Happiness	146
The 3 Main Reasons for Unhappiness	146
Step 6: Cultivate Nourishing Relationships	153
Step 7: Develop Healthy Lifestyle Habits	160
Eat Consciously	161
Be Mindful of Your Surrounding	162
Conclusion	**164**

Introduction

Congratulations on downloading this book and thank you for doing so. This book will help you in de-stressing your life and start living it on your own terms. It is a 7-step guide to simplify your life for a happy you.

Stress and anxiety have become an obvious and acceptable part of life these days. Our minds are so much cluttered with things that we are forgetting the ways to live happily. Stressful, complicated and mundane life is becoming a norm. This book will help you in dealing with this sorry state of affairs.

It will walk you through the ways in which stress is affecting our lives these days. It will give you insights on eliminating the stress from your daily lives. This book will specifically help you in relieving the physical and emotional symptoms of stress from life.

It will show you the ways in which you can reduce the decision fatigue and de-stress yourself.

This book will help you in understanding the impact of stress and anxiety on relationships. It will give you tips to reduce stress and anxiety in dating and relationships.

Toxic relationships add a high amount of stress to our lives. We all know it, but choose to ignore it. This degrades the quality of life and scars it. This book will help you in understanding the extent of stress these relationships can add and the ways to end them.

This book is your comprehensive guide to remove stress from your life and start living happily.

Our mind is simply amazing. There can be no other word that can better describe our mind. Either you are talking about the mind in terms of physiological wonders or its psychological prowess; it can do some pretty amazing stuff. It is full of immense possibilities and has unlimited capabilities. Yet, some people always feel rattled by their mind.

Commonly, people feel that their mind is never at peace. There is an incessant commotion inside the head. Some people believe that their mind is hyperactive. It is always up to something. There is an out of control banging of thoughts, random thoughts, weird thoughts, negative thoughts, or thoughts of helplessness. These thoughts leave people nervous, sad, worried, or distraught. They are never at peace with themselves. They are always agitated.

They think fuzzy and remain alarmed. They feel unfocused and disoriented.

These are all clear signs of a cluttered mind. A mind that is overworking and not thinking straight will become unproductive and will lead to several complex problems. Happiness will always evade people with such a mind. If you are also able to relate to these things, then this book is for you. It will help you in decluttering your mind and thinking rationally.

There are things that especially lead to a lot of mental clutter. This book will explain the main things that cause clutter in the mind and make life difficult. It will give you a framework to deal with such garbage for making your life simpler and happier.

Letting Go of the Baggage of the Past

We all carry some baggage of the past. It is inevitable. There are things that have been beyond our control or things have happened when we weren't very careful. However, the best thing about the past is that it is gone. The burden of the past can be as heavy or light as you want it to be. However, most people always carry the baggage of the past and let it influence their present. They are not able to let off the weight from their shoulders. Their leaves their judgment and actions impaired by the past. It is a cause of miseries in life. This book will help you in dealing with such baggage of past.

Dealing with Continuous Mental Chatter

The unremitting chatter going around in the mind is nagging. It is similar to the terrible and unnecessary honking of the horn unnecessarily. It renders you incapable of experiencing the true joys in life. The blissfulness in life is never there. It impairs your cognitive abilities. It slows you down and affects your decision-making abilities. It can also leave you confused, bewildered and absent-minded. This book will help you in understanding the reasons for this mental chatter and the ways to deal with it.

Avoiding Negative Thought Patterns

Have negative thoughts become your problem and affecting your abilities to process constructive thoughts? Do negative things easily drive your mind? Do fears and worries keep you on the edge? Are you always in the survival mode and you keep getting 'fight and flight' emotions from inside? These are all negative thought patterns. Negative thought patterns become a part of personality. They influence your thinking and actions. You start carrying an undesirable aura around yourself. This book will help you in dealing with negative thought patterns. It will help you in understanding the mechanism of negative thought patterns and the ways to break them.

Unlocking Happiness

Happiness is the most sought-after gift. There is no one in this world who doesn't want to be happy. Yet, we keep on feeling miserable without any solid reason. Our negative thought pattern is highly responsible for it. In place of counting the blessings, we spend our lives in counting the shortcomings. We forgo the simple joys in life and the right to be and feel happy without giving much thought. This book will help you in looking at happiness from a child-like perspective. It will help you in appreciating precious things in life to which we never pay any attention.

Cultivating Healthy Relationships

Relationships are a great source of joy. They provide the required support in life. They give meaning to happiness. However, cultivating nourishing relationships is always a problem for people with a cluttered mind. They are never able to focus on the priorities due to the overwhelming number of thoughts floating in their mind. You can learn a lot about forming strong relationships in this book.

Developing Healthy Habits

Our habits play a very important role in shaping our lives. Healthy habits make our lives simpler. They help in reducing the clutter in the mind and also from our surrounding. They ensure that you do the right things at the right time. However, developing healthy habits is always a difficult task for most. We always remain in a flux. This book will shed light on the ways to develop healthy habits for a more fulfilling life.

Life is supposed to be simple, joyful and meaningful. Being the most superior race on earth we must have a better time than other organisms. Yet, if you take a closer look, other organisms are having a gala time as compared to us. Their life is peaceful, content and a lot carefree. Our luxuries keep us confined. Excess of choices keeps us anxious. We feel more and more stressed.

Our mind has a very important role to play in it. The more cluttered it is, the less focus it can have on simplifying the life. We are in an endless pursuit to change others to suit us but care a little to change ourselves even a bit. This is the biggest problem we are facing today as a race. It keeps us stressed and anxious.

Our mind is always at work. On an average, the human mind has 25,000-50,000 thoughts in a day. It is very active and there is no problem so far. However, the problem is that 70% of these thoughts are full of negativity. So much negativity starts getting reflected in our personality. This begins an endless process of cover-ups and deceptions. One can never be happy in this scenario. To be really happy, the whole thought process would have to change. It not only affects your personality but also your relationships, actions, and physical health. A cluttered mind can make you unhappy and unhealthy.

This book will help you in dealing with the constant chatter going around in your mind. It will also give you easy and simple steps to declutter your mind so that you can simplify your life and learn to live happily.

This book will give you a 7-step approach to decluttering your mind to make life simple, easy and joyful.

With the help of the simple methods given in this book, you will be able to declutter your mind. You will have a better control over your thought process. You will be able to find joy even in simpler things and enjoy even smaller accomplishments in a bigger way. Your joy will not get sullied by frivolous things like contempt, jealousy, and competition. You will be able to take ownership of your happiness.

There are plenty of books on this subject on the market, thanks again for choosing this one! Every effort was made to ensure it is full of as much useful information as possible, please enjoy!

Chapter 1: Why Are We Stressed?

There is No Reason for So Much Stress

Modern life is full of comforts and there can be no doubt in that. We are living in the most peaceful times.

- Our days of being vulnerable prey are over. We dominate this planet.
- We have the technology by our side to do most of our jobs.
- The security of food is much greater these days. At least, the world is not worried that there'll be a widespread famine even if there are a few seasons of drought.
- There is no fear of the warring tribes.

- Terrible world wars are not claiming countless lives.

- Medical facilities are at their best ever. Never in the past medical science had been so advanced. From organ transplants to complicated medical procedures, the medical science ensures that most of the health problems get resolved as quickly and as painlessly as possible.

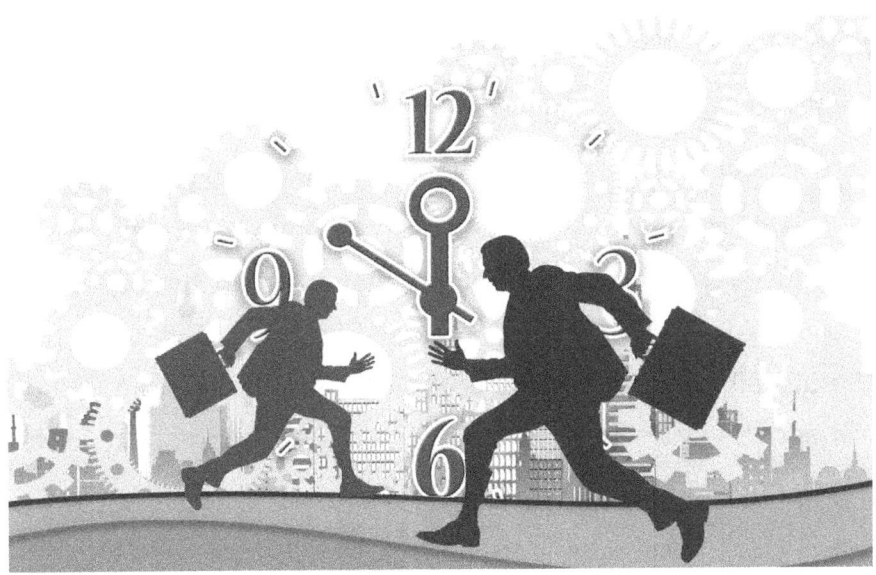

Stress in Daily Life is Real

However, despite all these facts, we are not at ease. Even the luxuries at our disposal have failed to reduce the level of stress and anxiety in our lives. In fact, we are the most stressed generation ever despite having no imminent threat to life. Statistics reveal that 73% of all working adults experience varying degrees of stress in their daily lives. Not the temptation to get a better package, but stress is the biggest reason for job change in the modern world. Even kids are suffering from a great deal of stress these days.

Stress, anxiety, and worries have become a common part of modern lifestyle. Our stress levels remain unusually high even in situations when there should be no stress at all. We need reasons to be happy. We have become naturally unhappy. This is the opposite of what should have been the norm. It is a very sad and depressing state of affairs.

Stress is a Natural Biological Response

In general, stress in itself has never been an alien or bad phenomenon for us. Our bodies have passed through thousands of years of evolution to learn to generate the stress response. Whenever we perceive any kind of threat, danger, or hostility, our body generates a stress response. This response creates an intense state of arousal to stimulate action. It is a very helpful defense mechanism. Without apt stress response, the survival of the human race wouldn't have been possible in a similar fashion. However, the problem is that now we are overdoing the stress response. We feel stressed even on things that do not need that level of concern.

One of the best things about modern life is that there are very few 'do or die' scenarios on a day-to-day basis. We aren't struggling for survival in the real sense. The competition at the workplace, the struggle to meet both ends meets, and social pressures aren't deadly in nature. Yet, our mind doesn't perceive them any less dangerous. We have given stress a completely new dimension.

Unusual Grounds for Stress

Ours is the most anxious, worried, and stressed out generation. It seeks stress and anxiety and when it doesn't get real things to worry about, it finds the unreal ones.

- We get intimidated by the happening life of our online friends and start feeling stressed. More often than not, social posts are presenting an unreal picture, and we know it. Yet, we remain stressed. Our mind remains cluttered. We keep feeling miserable.

- Simple choices in life can make us anxious. Ever felt anxiety in picking a cereal in a superstore? There is no reason to feel so, yet we keep questioning ourselves. We make simple decisions so important for ourselves.

- We keep aspiring for things that we don't even need. Success or failures shouldn't matter in such cases, but we make them a cause of stress.

- We let outside influence of news, social media and gossip affect our mind. Information overload is increasing the stress and we are allowing it to do so.

Stress is a normal phenomenon that our body can use to its advantage. However, the constant and unrealistically magnified perception of stress is very dangerous. It has deep ramifications on our physical, emotional, and psychological health.

A cluttered and confused mind can miscalculate the threats and increase stress levels unreasonably. Controlling stress is one of the most important requisites for a healthy, relaxed, and meaningful life

Chapter 2: Negative Impact of Stress on Your Health, Emotions, and Psyche

Stress Has Serious Impact

Stress, worry, and anxiety can make you physically unwell. From experiencing physical symptoms like pain, stiffness, indigestion, and insomnia to emotional symptoms like irritability, bad temper, and worthlessness, the impact of stress can be severe.

Neglecting the impact of stress can be dangerous. Stress leaves a strong impact on your health. It will be visible and will affect your personality and performance. You can try to hide the symptoms of stress, but this wouldn't negate its impact.

Some of the Physical Symptoms of Stress

Clumsiness in Attitude, Rash, and Accident Prone Behavior

Stress is a result of clouded thinking. You keep miscalculating things and then make last minute adjustments. This brings clumsiness in your behavior. Your decisions become rash and accident-prone. In most cases, these things happen when you try to bite more than you can chew. If you want to have everything in your plate at once, preventing the spilling gets difficult.

These days, people also try to give it the fancy name of multi-tasking. Our mind works best when it is focused on one thing at a time. Complete focus brings perfection. It reduces the chances of accidents and leads to better results. Your mind has a clear objective. It is the best way to deal with things. Taking one step at a time ensures that you are always on a strong footing and grounded. If you want to remove clumsiness from your attitude, clearing the clutter from your mind is very important.

Pain in Shoulders, Back, and Neck

Stress leads to some strange chemical reactions in our body. When you are stressed, alarmed, or anxious, your body starts releasing the stress hormones. These hormones create stiffness in your shoulders, neck, and back. These changes are designed to make you more resilient to damage in case of attack. They made us better equipped to handle combat situations. However, in modern life, stress is not caused due to physical danger, but as a result of worries and anxieties. It lasts longer as your mind stays fixed on that problem. Prolonged stiffness brought by these circumstances leads to stiffness and pain in shoulders, back, and neck.

The best way to deal with this problem is to take short breaks. Deviate your mind from the current problem and indulge your mind into something else. The more relaxed you feel, the fewer the problems would be.

Tensions and Headaches

Stress has a profound impact on our brain. When you are in stressful situations, your heart-rate increases, breathing quickens and your blood pressure rises. Your body starts pumping more blood and oxygen into your system to handle the problem. Prolonged exposure to this condition leads to the contraction of muscles which lead to headaches.

Your mind would become foggy and would not be able to think clearly in such situations. Taking breaks in such situations is the best resort.

Diarrhea or Constipation, Indigestion, Ulcers, or Heartburn

Your mind and the rest of your body may look separate but in reality, they are closely interconnected. Stress not only causes problems to your brain but also transfers the information to the cells in your body. Your gut has more neurons than your spinal cord. Your gut produces a lot of acid in stressful situations. It leads to indigestion, ulcers, diarrhea or constipation and heartburn.

Therefore, stress is not only a problem for your head but your gut too. If you are in a gut-wrenching situation or need to make a decision, which has put you in a fix, leave it aside for a few moments to cool down. Distracting yourself from the point for the moment helps in bringing clarity of thought.

Excessive Cravings for Stimulants like Caffeine, Cigarettes, and Change in Appetite

Excessive stress puts a heavy burden on your mind. It starts looking for stress relievers and this is where caffeine, cigarettes, chocolates come in play. These things led to the release of stress-relieving neurotransmitters called dopamine and serotonin. They make you feel better. However, overdependence on these things can lead to addiction and cause potential damage.

Abusing these things is a symptomatic treatment and will have no long-term advantage. The best way always is to address the cause of the problem. Your high-stress level is the main problem and until the reasons for high stress are not addressed, things won't change.

Disturbed Sleep, Insomnia, Nightmares

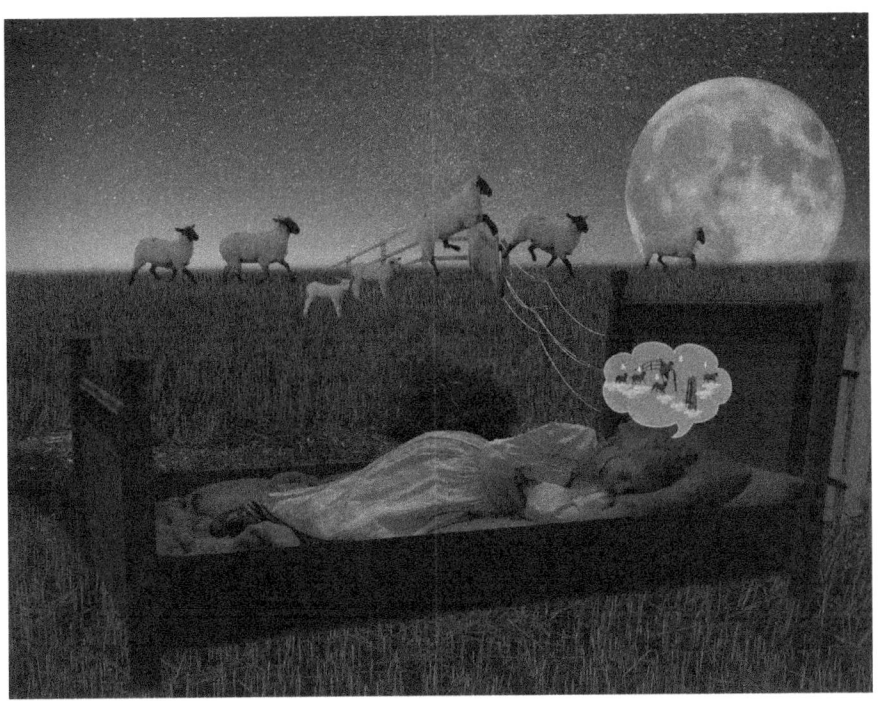

Sleep is one of the best stress busters. It helps your body in relaxing and releasing the stress. However, when your mind is not at rest, sleep is a luxury you can't afford. Stress has a strong impact on sleep patterns. People suffering from high stress have erratic sleep patterns and suffer from insomnia. If your mind is too much cluttered, your subconscious will keep playing the same scary scenarios even in your sleep and you can have nightmares.

This problem can only be resolved by consciously addressing the issues. The more you run away from the problem, the scarier they'll become. You should prepare yourself to address the issues in reality. Write down the problems you are facing in place of running them repeatedly in your mind. This clears some space in your mind and helps in removing the clutter. You can also discuss the problem with your family and friends as this gives the problem an outside perspective. Discussing it with others also helps you in coming out with a disclosure. The problems begin to scare you a bit less. If your stress is affecting your sleep, then you should start acting quickly as the problem would escalate pretty soon. It will also affect you physically as well as emotionally. You will feel more tired and foggy due to lack of sleep and will lose clarity of thought and energy.

Weight Gain

People normally associate weight gain with poor eating habits and bad food. However, abrupt weight gain also has its roots in high-stress levels. When you are under stress, your body releases a stress hormone called cortisol. This hormone sends your body in safe mode and most of the weight loss functions stop working efficiently. It is one of the strongest reasons for sad or depressed people exhibiting significant weight changes. Stress also leads to emotional and compulsive eating that also helps in weight gain.

A significant increase in weight due to stress will start a vicious cycle. It would make shedding weight difficult and cause more weight-related stress. If you are experiencing weight gain and feel that your stress is a reason behind it, then start taking preventive measures right away. Create healthy distractions for yourself. Walking, exercise, yoga, swimming, and other such physical activities will not only help you in burning more fat, but they'll also help in distracting your mind from the stress.

There are several other physical symptoms related to stress like low energy levels, acne, dry skin, frequent infections, substance, and drug abuse, and other addictions. All these things will keep pushing you in a corner towards more depression, anxiety, worries, and loneliness. Not attempting to get out of them isn't a solution.

Most of the stress is a result of cluttered thinking. Your mind stops thinking rationally or gets pinned down towards a wrong direction. A fresh start towards the problem can help in solving the problem. You can take a break from the problem.

Remember that stress doesn't only have physical symptoms but emotional ones too. It is working on your emotions too. The longer you remain under stress, the more difficult it will get to come out of it.

Some of the Emotional Symptoms of Stress

The Feeling of Being Overwhelmed

Problems can start looking overwhelming. It can feel like that they have pinned you down. Feeling helpless under them will be of no use. Try hard to overcome them. Use affirmations to remind yourself that you can come out of stressful situations and they aren't going to last long.

Feeling Sad or Hopeless

There will be times when the tunnel starts looking endless. However, everything has an end in the world, problems too. Feeling sad or helpless only makes winning more and more difficult.

Irritability

Stress causes irritability and that takes away your ability to rationalize. It is a bad move from all aspects. The more irritable you get, the more hostile and unreceptive environment you'll create for yourself. If you are becoming irritable, moving away from the problem for some time is the best solution.

The Feeling of Guilt and Worthlessness

Stress can lead to feelings of guilt and worthlessness. You will have to constantly remind yourself that the situation isn't permanent and it doesn't define you. Positive affirmations and indulgence in something creative is the best way to overcome these negative feelings.

Becoming Oversensitive

Stressful situations make people oversensitive to comments. This creates more negativity. Your thinking gets muddy and your decisions get mixed with ego. It is a negative response. Listening emphatically and understanding the situation is the right solution.

Procrastination

When you find something tough or challenging, the first response is to avoid it. However, in day-to-day life, there are many things that can't be passed on that easily.

People tend to delay such things indefinitely and that leads to more problems. Procrastination is a cognitive effect of stress. It is created by your flight response to the situation. Not dealing with the problem only decreases the time at hand to deal with it, but wouldn't dilute its intensity.

Ways to Get Relief from Physical Symptoms of Stress

Eat or Chew Something

There are scientific studies that reflect that chewing something or eating reduces the stress levels. It creates a temporary distraction. You can chew sugar-free gums or chew fruits to create a distraction from stress.

Do Yoga

Yoga has proven benefits in relieving physical stress. It helps in relaxing your muscles that also brings down your mental stress. The break from the problem and increased physical activity helps in relaxing you completely. If you are having a stressful routine, doing yoga for a few minutes in a day can be of great help.

Meditation

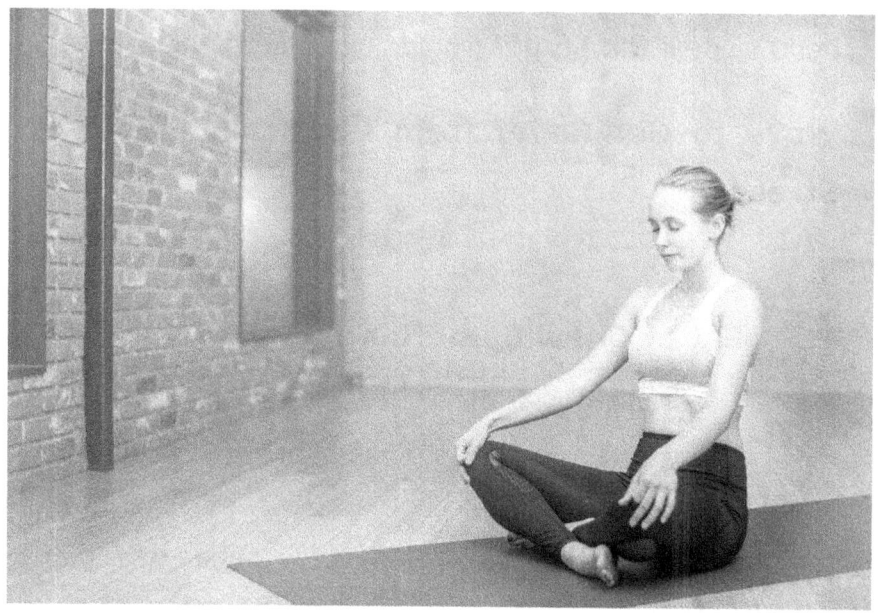

Meditation is one of the best ways to take off your brain from random thoughts and relax your brain. It helps you in self-introspection and also gives you an outsider view of the problem. Meditation has been known for reducing the stress levels to a great degree. The deep breathing routine in meditation especially helps in bringing more oxygen and releasing stress from the muscles. You can practice meditation for some time whenever you feel highly stressed. Practicing meditation daily in the morning or evening also helps in keeping your overall stress levels low.

Take a Break from Your Computer Screen

Prolonged and uninterrupted use of a computer is known for causing stress. It creates tension in the shoulder, neck, and back muscles. Your mind also becomes foggy and stops thinking sharply. If you are feeling stressed while working, you should take breaks at short intervals. This will lower the amount of physical stress.

Listen to Music

Music is a natural stress reliever. If you are feeling stressed, listening to your favorite music can help you a lot. Simply plug in the kind of music you like and give yourself a break.

Find Ways to Laugh

Laughter is one of the best ways to lower the physical stress levels in your body. You can watch funny videos or find something else that you find amusing.

Laughing even for a bit will have a profound effect on your stress level.

Maintain Distance from Social Networking Websites

Studies have proven that social networking websites like Facebook, Instagram, and Twitter make you feel sadder and less satisfied. They raise the levels of anxiety and do not add anything constructive. Staying away from social networking websites can help you in decreasing your stress levels.

Take Long Walks

Long walks have a very soothing impact. They give you the time to self-introspect and you tend to find better solutions after going for walks. They also raise the levels of hormones in your body that lower stress.

This list by no means is exhaustive. Everyone has personal triggers for stress and happiness. Find something that helps you in taking off your mind away from stressful situations. The important thing is to give yourself time to sort the things in your mind.

Stress is simply caused by the clouding of your mind. You have the ability to sort the problems you face. Only the temporary blinding of vision due to an overwhelming problem leads to cloudy thinking. You can sort it by giving yourself some time to think over it.

Living with stress is the worst option that we can choose but unfortunately, we all have made it our primary choice. The most disturbing part is that we want to remain completely unmindful of the fact. There is a widespread deniability and it is making the situation even worse.

Stress is a Result, Not the Cause

Stress is causing a lot of problems. We all want to get rid of this stress and live a relaxing life. A whole new industry has sprung which is trying to ease stress. But, is it effective? The answer is a resounding 'No'. It is trying to treat the symptoms and not the causes.

Stress is simply a consequence of our misplaced priorities, unfulfilled desires, and negative thought patterns.

The real cause of the problem is our Cluttered Mind. By the time, you do not sort your aspirations, goals, and priorities, the problems would remain in place.

Decluttering of the mind is crucial for getting actual relief from stress. When your mind is clear, you'll have better goals. Your aspirations from life would be more definite and rewarding. You will not succumb to the pressure and will have better ways to handle it.

If you really want to lead a stress-free life, then you will have to learn the ways to manage your life more successfully. You cannot achieve this goal until and unless your mind starts to think clearly.

Chapter 3: Declutter Your Mind for Reducing Stress

Clearing of the mental clutter is the only sustainable way to have a stress-free and meaningful life. When your mind is in a position to think clearly and make decisions based on priorities rather than instincts, your life becomes easier.

These days, the stress in life has increased so much that people have started thinking that peace is the goal of life, it isn't. Peace is the way of life and leading a meaningful and constructive life should be the goal. Even the animals and birds that do not have the same cognitive abilities as ours lead a peaceful life. There is no reason for this life to not be peaceful or be chaotic until some external force is applied.

Think of young kids for that matter. They lead a peaceful and happy life. You need to apply force to make them unhappy. They are beaming with life. But, as we grow, we become gloomy, stressful, and sad. The person doesn't change. It is the clutter that gets accumulated in mind and brings the change in attitude.

If you closely look at the life of a child:

- A child has easy goals
- A child has clear priorities that bring happiness
- A child has easy decisions to make
- A child has few things to compete for

As you grow all these things change for you. You set unrealistic goals for yourself. Your priorities are complex and most of the times have no bearing in present. The number of choices in your life increase causing a lot of indecisiveness. This leads to anxiety, unhappiness, and stress. You increase the competition for yourself. Your mind starts raising the bar on its own. The more cluttered your mind is, the tougher your life will get.

The reason for most of our stress is unconscious decision taking. It is a result of a cluttered mind where decisions are mostly based on trends or instincts. Becoming mindful of our decision-making process and decluttering the mind can help in solving most of these problems.

We are more focused on living a full life rather than living a fulfilling life. We are running in a mindless race to gather material possessions not knowing their use or worth once we have gained them. We waste our lives running after success only to realize in the end that it wasn't worth the pain anyway.

We work for numerous hours in offices. We sacrifice our precious time in looking at the files and miss the smiles blooming on the lips of our toddlers. This is a great loss that can have no compensation in terms of monetary gains.

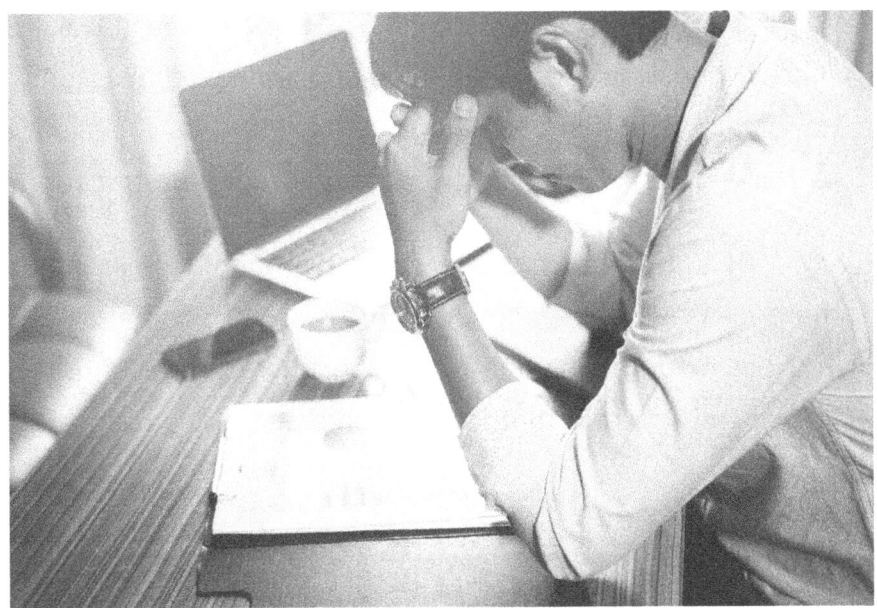

We bear great stress in form of responsibilities. We slog for endless hours in jobs, only to realize that we don't even have the necessary passion for the job. All these things increase stress in life. These are mindless activities are carried out without giving much thought.

This endless talk about not focusing on work and career entirely for money or searching for passion may look a little offbeat. To a materialistic mind, it is a bit off the track. However, it doesn't make the fact any less sad that we are ready to exchange happiness and joy in life in exchange for stress and worthless material possessions.

You work day and night to get rich. You have more than 1 home, more than 1 car and money that is only of any value to you in bank statements. But, you are skeptical to work for something that can give you real gratification.

If you think that searching for happiness in place of material wealth is a difficult and absurd phenomenon, then you are wrong. Not only a person but a whole nation has shown to the world that it is possible and holds merit.

Curious Case of Bhutan

Bhutan is a small landlocked country in South Asia. It shares its borders with China and India. This country has the concept of Gross National Happiness (GNH).

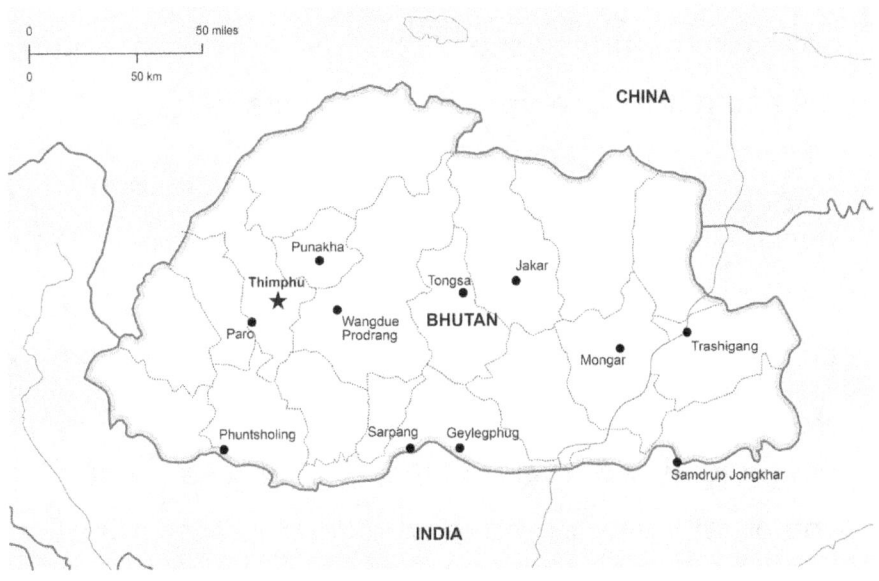

It means that it measures its success in terms of happiness of its citizens. Rest of the world has a different and very common parameter and that is Gross Domestic Product (GDP). The worth of a nation is accounted for by the number of goods it produces. No wonder, the most successful countries in the world have the highest stress level rates.

Robert F. Kennedy in his speech in 1968 had said that GDP measures everything in short, except that which makes life worthwhile. If you look at it, most of the developed nations are battling with high-stress rates. In the US and Canada alone, the stress rates are above 70%. The European countries also do not have a very promising statistics.

On the other hand, Bhutan, a small country that doesn't have too many industries or trade links. Yet, it has a happiness rate of 48.7%. This means that almost half of the population in that country is happy with whatever it has. The country focuses on the psychology of well being, time use, education, community vitality, ecology, diversity, acceptance, and happiness quotient.

If keeping the people happy, satisfied, and passionate can be the goal of a nation, it couldn't be too difficult for an individual to ensure personal happiness.

The math to remain happy isn't very complicated. You only need to remove the clutter from your mind. Leave everything aside that holds no meaning to you.

There are some major areas that have a deep impact on your happiness. If things are neglected in these areas, they automatically lead to stress. Prioritize and see the things you want to have in these areas:

Health

While planning for life, most people never even give a fleeting glance at the health. While we are young, we take it for granted that we'll always be young, healthy, happy and energetic. This notion precipitates pretty fast and we have nothing else to do other than sulk. Health is one of the most important factors that affect our happiness and stress. If you are consciously planning for a stress-free life then leaving health out of that plan is an injustice.

Chart out a definite plan for health and fitness. Decide the amount of time and effort you want to give to remain healthy.

Career

We spend the highest amount of time and energy at our workplace. We study, learn, and gain experience in order to have a stable and rewarding career. But, what use is a career that only keeps you aggravated and dissatisfied? It may give you the money, but that money is only good for boosting your ego and buying stress relievers.

A career should always be rewarding. Something that fuels your passion so that you can become more productive. Do not choose a career that makes you feel miserable. It will make you a part of the rat race.

Work is an important part of life. Yet, it is only a part of life and not the whole of it. If you start compromising with your life for work, in the end, you'll be left with very few things to remain happy. Your work life must have a balance. The amount of work you take must be based on the amount of work you can do. Succumbing to peer pressure, competition and greed may snatch away your happiness.

Relationship

Relationships are important as they complete us. They bring a sense of inclusion in life. However, expectations in relationships and especially unrealistic expectations can turn them toxic. Have a clear idea about the things you want in a relationship. Have a clear, frank and open dialogue about it while entering into a committed relationship. Be more open, accepting and inclusive.

Family

The family is something we easily push aside while making important decisions. The family has its place in life and it should be clear in your mind while you make your decisions.

Self-Improvement

The best thing about us human beings is that we have an indefinite potential for improvement. We can learn new things, languages, arts, craft and make ourselves better. Continuously work on making yourself better. Either it is developing your personality or learning new things, it will make you feel more satisfied. Nothing gives a greater sense of joy than the accomplishment of learning new things. It will keep stress low in your life.

Life Planning

Security is important in life to alleviate unnecessary stress. Planning for life reduces mental clutter. Things move in a more organized manner. You get more time to devote to yourself rather than worrying about the unknown contingencies. Plan things like budget, work, retirement, etc. well in advance.

Recreation

Enjoyment has a special place in life. It gives you joy and pleasure. The end goal of most of the above pursuits is to ultimately bring joy to your life. You must always have space for leisure in life. Plan recreational activities as you plan your work and budget. The moment you start neglecting recreation, stress starts going up.

Decide the Way You Really Want to Spend Your Time

Do not move with the herd. You must consciously decide the way you spend your time. If you feel that the time spent on watching TV is unproductive then it should be discontinued. Invest that time in more pleasurable activities. Stop watching the things or programs that add stress to your life. If watching violence or negative news disturb you, stay away from it. Mindless absorption of negativity for the sake of it is a leading cause of stress. This is what social media websites and TV does to you. They put you at the receiving end of the information for which you are not prepared. You do not have much control over the kind of information you will get.

If you like comedy and that makes you happy, then selectively watch comedy. Do not even get force-fed tragedy or thrillers by the TV or the internet.

Become Conscious of Earning and Spending Money

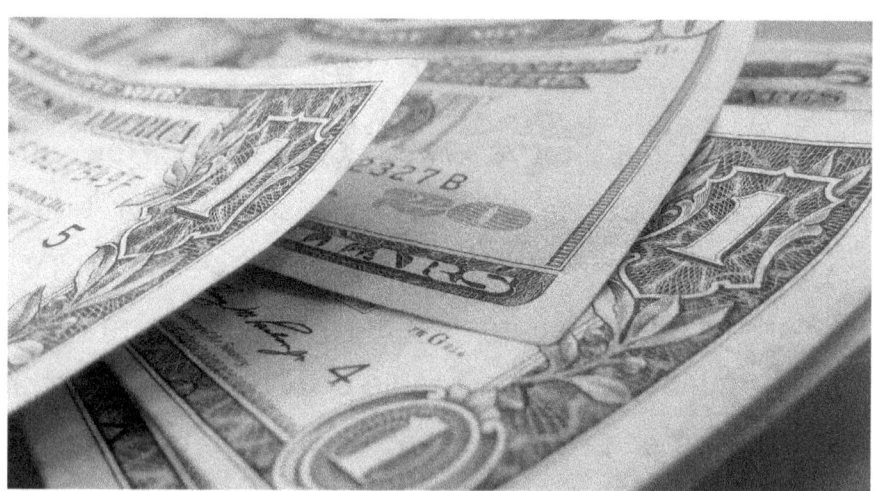

Both earning as well as spending money can increase your stress levels. The more you spend, the more you will become a slave of work. Spending doesn't mean more happiness. Stop identifying your happiness with your spending abilities. Learn to live with a bare minimum. This will increase the chances of happiness for you.

Cherish Moments

Most importantly, start appreciating life for its merits. Find time to praise life, nature and all the things that fill you with happiness. If you like something, then take out time to look at it more attentively. If anything attracts you, then pursue it.

Living life consciously is the beginning of starting your journey towards leading a stress-free life. Remain mindful of the life around you.

Chapter 4: The Role of Habits in Reducing Stress and Mind Clutter

Clutter at the physical, emotional, or psychological level causes stress. It is one of the biggest reasons for stress.

The physical clutter is obvious. Any excess material that's of no use to you is clutter. Anything that may have been used a long time ago but hasn't been put to use for more than a year is clutter.

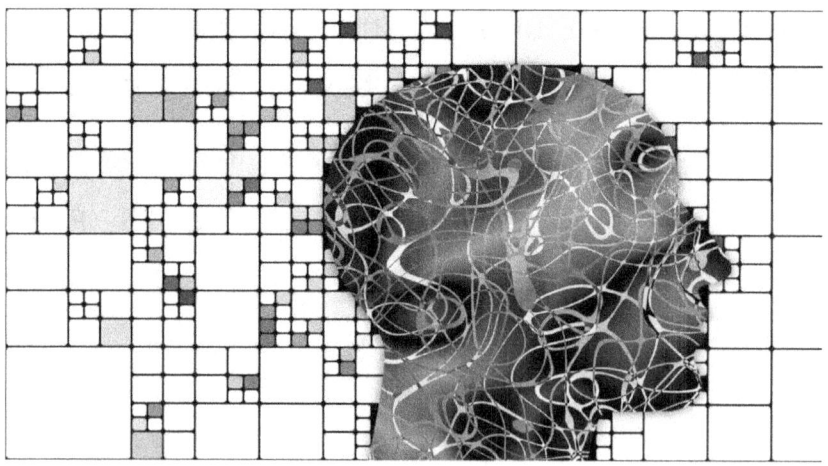

Clearing Physical Clutter is Easy

Clutter takes up space and energy. It uses up your productive energy and distracts you. Your focus can keep deviating if there is clutter around you. Clutter always reminds you that there is one job left to be sorted and you haven't done it. It has a great impact on your functioning and efficiency. You can sort physical clutter by simply removing the unnecessary items from your vision. You can make the system and workplace leaner and things would be better.

More Decision Making Means More Mental Clutter

However, things are not as easy with mental clutter. Our mind is processing thoughts 30 times faster than the fastest supercomputer in the world. It handles more than 1016 processes in a second. Even when you are not really thinking about it, your mind is continuously taking decisions.

For instance, take lunch one afternoon:

You are still in your cubical punching keys on your computer. But, as soon as your mind gets a fragrance of food, it starts thinking about it. The mind doesn't think in a restrained manner. It goes full throttle.

There are thoughts of things you want to eat at lunch, you would want but can't have. Would you be able to get a specific item in the lunch? Would it taste good? Would someone accompany you?

Most of the times, you are not even paying attention to it. Your active participation isn't even required. Your mind is capable of thinking all these in-between things. However, one thing that makes this a problem is that this thinking requires decision making. There are choices to be made.

Whenever there are choices to be made, your mind gets stuck. This activity requires your active participation. The mind wouldn't simply stop at giving you the choices but would question your decisions. This creates a dilemma and any kind of dilemma or hesitation will lead to mental clutter.

You are making thousands of such insignificant decisions in your day. Your mind keeps coming at the points where it requires a decision. It questions those decisions. It debates on the success or failure of those decisions. All this leads to the generation of mental clutter. Any kind of clutter will bombard your mind with excessive stimuli. Your mind would go on an overdrive. There will be unnecessary distraction and hesitation. There will be the physical, mental, and emotional stress of making such decisions. Your mind constantly keeps receiving messages that there is still work pending. It never comes to rest leading to fatigue. It creates anxiety and you may also feel the guilt or repentance of taking decisions. It inhibits your creativity, productivity, and problem-solving abilities. Countless activities of similar nature are running in the background.

All this leads to stress. If it continues for long, it converts into chronic stress and takes a toll on health. This is the reason people sitting at the position of great power start looking haggard and aged much earlier.

Let us consider this through the analogy of senior management in a company. The CEOs, presidents, and senior management people take fat paychecks while all the hard work is done by the lower level employees. It always looks unjustified. However, no one looks at the amount of decision making stress these people have to bear. The onus of taking the decision will come to them. They will be liable for those decisions. They will have to take responsibility for things over which they could exercise no control.

In a similar fashion, we also need to make several decisions in a day. Such minor and major decisions create some amount of clutter that will lead to stress. If you want to have a stress free life, then your focus should always remain on reducing such clutter.

The fewer number of decisions you have to make in a day, the lower the amount of mental clutter will be.

This is among the primary reasons that the most affluent people in the world keep their usual options simple.

Mark Zuckerberg, the CEO of Facebook wears the same color of clothes to work daily. He says that it saves the trouble of making choices every day. Barack Obama had all his suits of only two colors. He believed that reducing the number of things to choose from helped in easing the brain so that he could fully use it for decisions of great importance.

Habits That Help You in Reducing the Mind Clutter

The Oxford dictionary says that habits are settled regular tendencies or practices, especially the ones that are hard to give up. This means that if you bring something into regular practice, it becomes your second nature. You can do it even without paying any attention to it. If you adopt healthy habits, you will have fewer things to worry about and your mind will be at pretty much ease. There will be much less stress to handle originating from taking decisions.

If we consider the earlier analogy once again, you'll find that lower level employees in an organization have to deal with much less stress.

Undoubtedly, lower level employees have to do very hard labor. They do not earn much but at the end of the day, but they have to make only simple choices. They are relatively leading a very low-stress life. They can sleep with peace in their homes while the CEO's roll restlessly in their plush homes.

You can also bring down the level of stress in your life by reducing the number of choices you have to make in a day. Adopting some good habit automates life and it becomes easier.

You will have less stress of making choices in daily life. It is either getting up in the morning or choosing the type of clothes you like to wear. From buying the groceries to the type of food you eat. Simpler habits will result in lower stress.

Chapter 5: Ways to Avoid Decision Fatigue

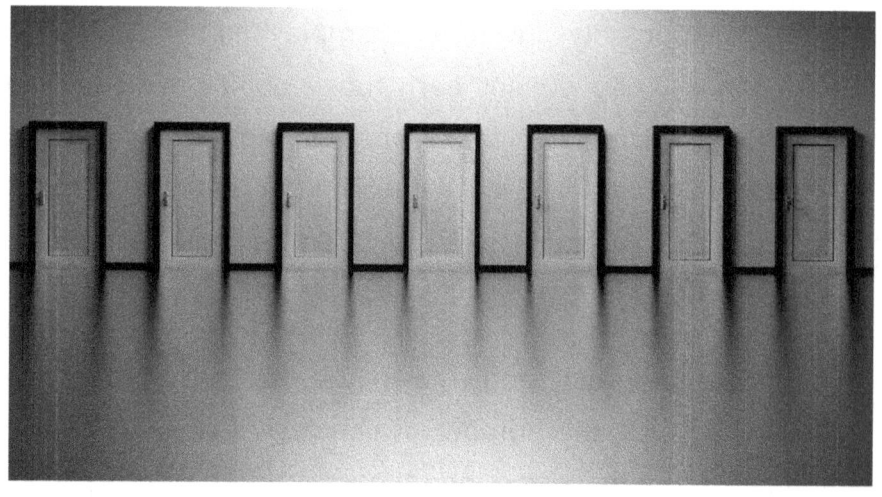

On an average, we make 35,000 conscious or unconscious decisions every day. Most decisions do not need your active involvement. However, even some simple decisions can cost you a lot of time and cause stress. A quick glance at an online sale can cost you an hour. Making the choice of breakfast can be tough for some people. To sleep or to go for a walk can be a harassing dilemma. These decisions can cause decision fatigue. They can make you feel exhausted, spent, or apathetic.

The best way to avoid facing decision fatigue is to follow some simple steps:

Build Habits into Your Schedule

Bringing habits into your schedule is the best way to avoid such decision-making points. If you have a fixed schedule that you follow, then such worries wouldn't arise. Fix a time for daily activities. Following a schedule keeps you sharp and makes you more efficient. It also eliminates the chances of procrastination from your life.

Be firm be firm

The dilemma of whether you are choosing the best or not can be crunching. However, most of the times it is a baseless debate. If there is a product, it is made for the consumption of someone. Do not look for the best qualities in the products, look for the qualities that you desire and once you find them, stick to your decision. Indecisive people radiate a lot of negativity.

Make Joy and Happiness the Parameter for Your Decisions

The final deciding parameter of most of the things should be the amount of joy it would bring in life. We all have this as the end goal behind all our decisions. However, mostly this is hidden behind riders. If I buy a bigger TV than John, I would have an edge and that would make me happy. This is a bad decision process. John can buy an even bigger TV at any point and then my same TV would start making me feel miserable. If you are going to buy a TV, then the only correct question is the kind of TV that would make you really happy. The kind of viewing experience you would want. The amount of clarity you are looking for. The size that would fit your wall and suit your room size. Your joy and happiness should be directly behind your decisions and not some

hidden agenda. It would take away the decision fatigue.

Choose a Role Model

Following a role model is always easy when you are picking such habits. It makes your choices simple. If you have a role model then put them in your place for easy and stress-free decision making. Imitating their decisions will absolve you of all the responsibility and fatigue. The ultimate goal of the practice is to ensure that you have to make a fewer number of such decisions on a daily basis.

You do not have to lose your identity. It is only for taking decisions that have no effect on the course of your life. In fact, easy decision-making process frees up a lot of time for you. You will be in a better position to ponder over the larger problems in a relaxed manner.

Learn to Say 'No'

Being resolute is very important for the success of any such exercise. Despite your efforts, there will be times when you'll be standing at the crossroads.

You'll have to learn to firmly make a decision and go with it. You may not have the clarity but if you keep fighting with the idea, it will lead to stress. Learn to live by your decisions.

Some Simple Stress Saving Habits

Eating Similar Food

Food is an important choice that we make every day. You have several meals a day. If you start spending 10-15 minutes before every meal to decide the menu, you are doing a great disservice to yourself and humanity. You are only useful for the food producing industry. The best way to expedite the process, or to make it simple is to either plan in advance for the week or month or eat similar food daily. You can have minute variations but stick to the same script. This will save a lot of time and effort.

Have a Smaller Wardrobe

Trim your wardrobe as much as possible. The lower the number of choices in clothes you have, the shorter you'll take to get ready. It will save time and you wouldn't have to ponder about your shining armor daily. Limited choice of clothes is a strategy adopted by some of the most successful people in the world.

Follow Daily Routines

Follow daily routines like a clockwork. If you are being lenient about your routines then you are cheating yourself. Stick to the routines as they help in the formation of rigid habits. Look at the people retiring from military service. They need to train daily in the morning for around two decades. It is a compulsion in the beginning. But, they find it hard to shun the habit even after they have retired. The routine becomes a part of their life. It keeps them fit and functioning.

Have Fixed Corners in Your Schedule

Do not compromise with the time of separate activities. Everything has a definite importance in life. If you have designated a specific time of the day to one activity, do not try to fit the other into it. This adjustment trains your mind to make a compromise. It also has to make an unnecessary decision. Strictly avoid it in all circumstances.

If Something Makes You Feel Anxious, Drop It

Do not do things that cause stress. Modern life mandates us to do several things in peer pressure. This is tiring and uninspiring. If you do not like anything, learn to stay away from it. It will cause unnecessary levels of stress and anxiety which you had been trying to avoid in the first place.

Do Not Fall in the Trap of Problem of Choice

Economists say that the biggest problem of this world is not poverty or hunger; it is the problem of choice. Rich or poor, man or woman, healthy or sick, we all have to face this problem. We have to make numerous decisions on a daily basis. Some decisions make you feel liberated and others crush you down. The marketing industry has perfected the art of using the problem of choice to its advantage. They put you in the trap of choosing between better and worse, small and big, cheap and costly, bright or dull, light or heavy and in the process you end up making choices that were not even required. Keep your choices simple if you want to remain happy and stress-free for the whole of your life.

Chapter 6: Relationships and Stress

Stress has become such a common phenomenon that it has crept into every aspect of life these days and relationships are also not an exception. Relationships are meant to be an anchor. They provide moral, social, and emotional support. We look towards them for help. However, these days, relationships need more help than anything else in the world.

Stress in relationships is very common. We can see stress at every stage of a relationship. Either it is the dating stage, try to remain committed or breaking apart from a relationship, stress is omnipresent.

Of all the other things, stress in relationships is a dangerous phenomenon because if it exceeds too much, the connecting fiber of the society would get endangered. Therefore, it is very important that you try to maintain healthy relationships. In case, remaining in a relationship is not very viable, breaking apart in an amicable way in a timely manner is also very important.

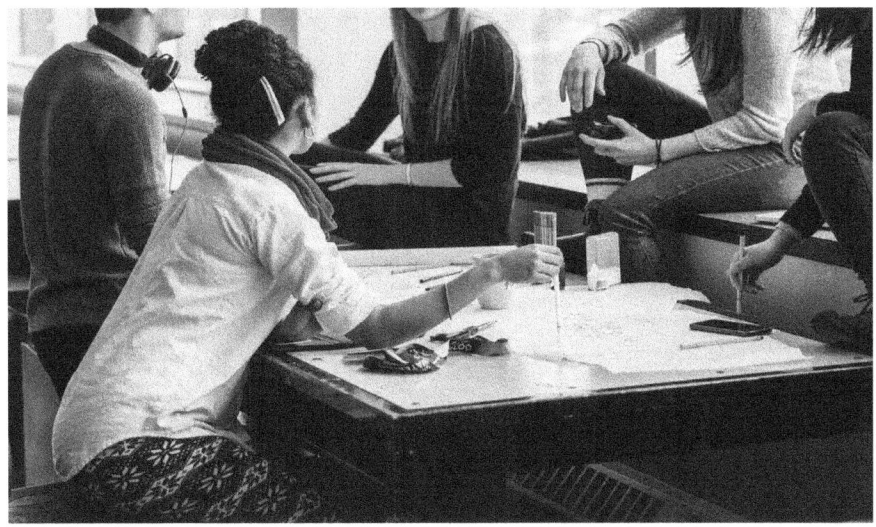

Relationships should never be taken lightly. Relationships are meant to compliment you. We cannot be everything at once and that's why we seek relationships to feel complete. They fill the void. Treating relationships in a frivolous manner is a serious mistake. You should take all the steps to make a relationship work as it takes time and energy to cultivate nourishing relationships.

The next three chapters will discuss the following:

1. Stress and anxiety in dating and the ways to lower it.

2. Things that lead to stress in relationships and the ways to deal with them.

3. Strategies to improve or eliminate bad relationships.

Chapter 7: Understanding and Dealing with Anxiety in Dating

Entering into a new relationship is not a very easy thing. Two different individuals with unique personalities need to accept each other. They have to acknowledge each other's strengths and weaknesses and learn to live with them. Put aside some of the differences in personalities and adapt. It is a fairly complicated procedure. Studies and age-old wisdom have taught that no amount of extended companionship can make two individuals one. Only those relationships survive the best that understand weaknesses of the partners and show inclusiveness. However, this is a learning process and takes time to develop. Dating is a completely different ballgame altogether. It is almost jumping into the pond without any idea of the depth.

Stress and anxiety in such cases are natural. Some people perfect their game with time and feel completely normal. Otherwise, stress and anxiety in dating are as common as yolk in an egg.

If you are worried about dating. Having the gut-wrenching feeling and developing the fight or flight response, then hold your horses a little bit more. You are not all alone in the boat.

It is Very Common

More than 18% of adult US population faces anxiety disorders. Roughly more than 15 million people are suffering from it. So, if you are feeling anxious, it is common. Even the people who are not suffering from any kind of anxiety disorder feel stressed, worried, and anxious about dates. There is no reason for you to not be alarmed. Getting to know, understand, and like a person is a big thing. It involves commitment, adjustments, and the works.

Most people think that throwing cheesy lines, looking confident, or being experienced can make a difference in the dating game. They completely ignore the aspect that the other person would also be going through the same feelings.

If you are new to dating, remain calm. It is not a gladiatorial conquest. You are going to know a new person. The more apprehensive you are, the tougher the knowing process will get. Remain calm and relaxed. If you are nervous, stressed, anxious or worried go easy on yourself.

Do not try to excessively hide it as it can make you defensive or even cocky.

Treat it as a similar experience for the other person and try to be as normal as possible. There is no race and you would eventually get to know each other.

It Can Make You Go Around in Circles and Feel Dumb

Anxiety usually makes the initial conversation difficult. Stammering, loss of words, temporary memory loss, the feeling of sheer stupidity are some common symptoms people feel. If you are also feeling the soon, then believe me it isn't a 'Eureka' moment. Most of the dating population feels the same way. Most probably the other partner is also going through the same experience. It wouldn't put a dent in your efforts.

You should continuously start to relax and keep the conversations to normal. Start with light chit-chat and see where the conversation takes you.

However, if you feel really stressed about the whole dating game and want to make things work, you can follow the points given below.

The Ways to Overcome Anxiety in Dating

Don't Hide the Facts

Deception can make your fears turn real. Dating is not about hiding, but about sharing. Deception is the worst strategy to be used in dating. When you are dating someone, exaggerating things, not disclosing important things about yourself, or lying can prove to be dangerous. It forms a wrong impression on the partner. It can start the relationship on a false foundation that is bound to fall.

If you are afraid to tell the truths about yourself due to the fear of rejection, then you are making a mistake. Relationships are close affairs. Your partner will get to know everything eventually. Getting to know things at a later stage lead to worse results. In a new relationship, you have very little to lose. However, this would change as the relationship matures. The emotional and psychological bonding would strengthen with time. If your partner gets to know the real truths then and decides to leave on the basis of those facts, it would hurt more.

Don't Judge or Fear of Getting Judged

People are excessively afraid of getting judged by the other partner in dating. However, they don't realize that while they fear getting judged, they are judging the dating partner themselves. Dating is more about knowing each other and not judging. If you are trying to enter into a relationship, then keep your prejudices aside and get to know the other person. Lower your guard and let the other person also know you better. This is the only way a new relationship can blossom. Keep your fears and anxieties aside.

Practice Acceptance

Unconditional acceptance of the qualities and shortcomings of a new partner is the best way to begin a relationship and sustain it.

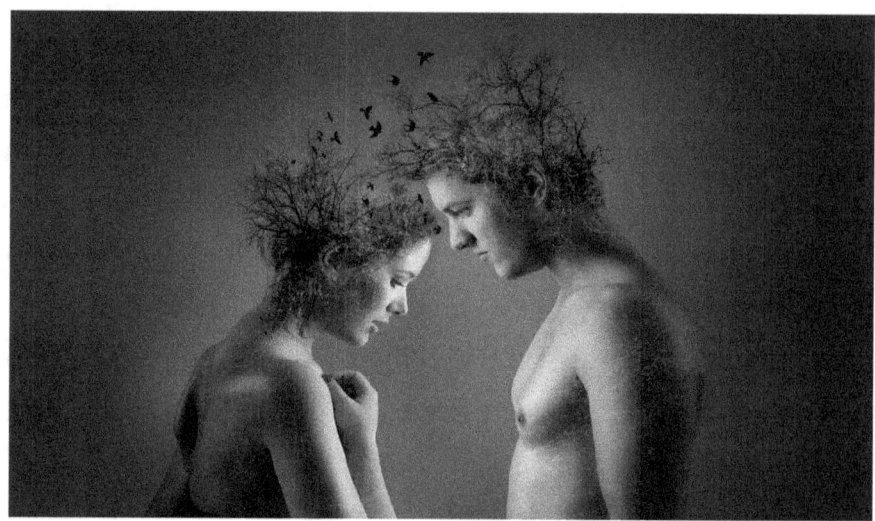

A relationship must always be inclusive. The relationships which are based on the merits and demerits of the partners do not last long. No one likes to be corrected at each and every step. If you are trying to do that with your partner, you should brace yourself for a big collision.

It's Not the End of the Road

People who treat dating as a once in a lifetime chance tend to fare far worse than those who treat it normally. Fear is bad for any kind of relationship. Such an emotion can make you look desperate and creepy. It is no way to treat a new relationship especially the one about which you know nothing. Enter into a relationship with an open mind. Give it your best effort and try to be honest and open. Do not go overboard with your efforts as it can make the other partner uncomfortable.

Live in the Present

Relationships are meant to bring joy in life. It is not the extent of the relationship but the amount of joy it brings in life. Joy comes in various packages. In the beginning look for the things that give joy to you. Once you start liking the relationship, you will put your best efforts to make it work and the same goes for the other partner too. Live the moment and try to rejoice it.

Chapter 8: Things That Lead to Stress in Relationships

There are many factors that can lead to stress in a relationship. Lack of understanding and acceptance is among the biggest reasons for stress and anxiety in a relationship. Mistrust and accusing behavior is also a big reason that leads to stress and eventual failure of a relationship.

It is important that you understand the factors that can create rifts in a relationship and sincere efforts should be put to mend the cracks. It is important to understand that no relationship is perfect. Relationships can never be perfect. They are always variable. There is always the space for adjustments and repair. If you can understand the problems in a relationship on time, such problems can be solved amicably.

Things That Lead to Stress in Relationships

Uncertainty About the Relationship

Uncertainty in the minds of partners in a relationship can creep anytime. They are not baseless as your behavior leads to such uncertainties a great extent. The important thing is to resolve the issues in time that have led to such uncertainties.

If you or your partner is having these thoughts then there is a serious need to have the commitment talk. Such concerns lead to high levels of stress and cloud the judgment and rational thinking. Reassurance of the commitment can work as an antidote in such scenarios.

Personal Insecurities

Partners can have insecurities. Most of the times, these insecurities are based on past experiences but they have a great impact on the present. Intentional or unintentional sarcasm, criticism or any judgment passed without much thought can also lead to such suspicions. Relationships are meant to be strong and supportive; however, they are attached with the thin threat of common trust and respect. Belittling, ridiculing or passing comments can put a huge dent in the relationship. If you or your partner is having such thoughts then it would be appropriate to have a thorough discussion over the subject.

Power Equation

For a relationship to go strong, both the partners should have their say in it. Domination by any one partner can leave the relationship off-balance. Balancing the power equation in a relationship is a tightrope walk. Relationships are not about exercising power but not having the power can make the partner feel vulnerable. Reassuring the partner of your sincerity and receptiveness is the right way to go at it.

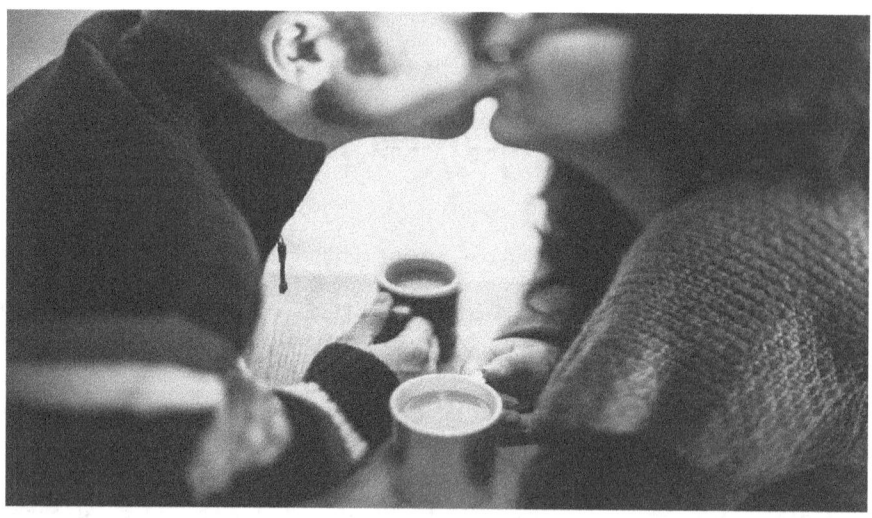

Lack of Boundaries

Boundaries are important in all kinds of relationship. When one partner starts to exceed their boundaries, the friction starts taking place. You must ensure that your partner gets the space he or she deserves and desires. Overstepping the boundaries can create distrust in relationships. Both the partners must always feel welcomed in a relationship and it cannot happen until they respect the set boundaries. A breach of boundary leads to stress and anxiety.

Safety Concerns

A relationship is a safe sanctuary. The role of the partners is to make each other feel safe and cared for in the relationship. Aggression in behavior and abusiveness can raise deep safety concerns. It raises the stress and anxiety levels astronomically. If you or your partner is feeling anything of this sort, you should talk to each other or take professional help. Ignoring such concerns will only lead to an abrupt end of the relationship.

Communication Gap

Healthy communication is the backbone of any relationship. It ensures that both the partners are able to raise their concerns and express themselves clearly. Lack of proper communication should always be taken seriously. If your communication channel with your partner has broken, you should put efforts to mend it back. Without proper communication, partners cannot raise their concerns. It increases the stress, anxiety, and suffocation in any relationship and makes it toxic.

Blame Game

The blame game is the most undesirable kind of communication in any relationship. It blocks the chances of improvement and puts the other partner in a defensive position. Relationship woes are meant to be addressed in a more civilized manner. Resorting to blame game can end the possibility of any future improvement, recovery, or reconciliation. It raises the threat perception to a whole new level. It also stimulates the fight or flight response in the partners.

Unloading of Past

Human brains have a vast storage capacity. They can record almost everything. However, in case of any kind of dispute between the partners in a relationship, only the bad memories come back in a flash. It is one of the most disastrous things to wipe out all the good deeds of the partner and start counting the sins. It leads to mistrust and animosity. Partners should reconcile their differences in a civilized manner where they should discuss the areas of improvement and work on them. Unloading the past only brings back the baggage of the past in present.

Maintaining a relationship is a delicate job. A relationship is a union of two separate identities. It is in nature for two unique individuals with a separate set of qualities to have an attraction for each other. However, their uniqueness can also lead to friction. The trick is to run the whole thing in a synchronized manner.

Healthy relationships can help in lowering the stress and anxiety levels as they make you feel loved, wanted and cared for. They make you feel the connection and the longing. However, the same relationships can also increase the stress levels if they are not handled with care or not treated properly.

You must give your best to any relationship. It is the foundation of a healthy life. Our society is entirely based on relationships. But, you should never forget the fact that every attempt has an endurance level. If you ever feel that your relationship is not fulfilling anymore or is bringing more stress to life than joy, then ending such relationships in an amicable way is the best resort.

Chapter 9: Strategies to Improve or Eliminate Bad Relationships

Some things in life go beyond the stage of repair. The friction in some relationships increases so much that it is best to end them and start fresh. These relationships simply become toxic. They add more and more stress, worries, sorrows and panic in life. They drain your mental energies and degrade your mental health.

A relationship means an exchange of love and emotions between two individuals. It is a lot like trade, only here your feelings, emotions, and values are at stake. A broken relationship causes a lot of pain and discomfort. But, sometimes it becomes impossible to have a positive perspective about some relationships. The pain and turmoil in such relationships increase so much that it is best to let them go.

Unfortunately, many people are not even able to determine the extent where a relationship becomes toxic. They keep trying to revive it beyond the point of repair. Such efforts keep increasing the agony and bear no fruits. They cause exasperation, feeling of defeat and deceit. They hurt a lot and you, unfortunately, had invested a lot of emotions in them. However, like a gangrene infected limb, it is always in your larger interest to let it go. The more they cling to you, the more they'll fill you with stress, negativity, disappointment, bias, and pain.

Some of the Symptoms of Such Toxic Relationships

Abusiveness: The relationships that have become physically, verbally, and emotionally abusive. These relationships become dangerous and can cause serious damage to you physically as well as emotionally.

Lack of Integrity: The relationships that involve deceit and dishonesty or lack of integrity become highly toxic. Such relationships erode the fabric of trust. If you try to remain in such relationships for long, you'll find it difficult to trust anyone in the future.

Incompatibility: Relationships also become toxic due to severe incompatibility issues. Living with such people becomes an eternal torture. You find it more and more challenging to cope with them intellectually, emotionally or physically.

Mental Incapacity: Relationships with partners having untreated mental health issues. Such relationships can get dangerous as your partner will not have the intellectual integrity to make correct decisions.

Addictions: Relationships with people falling prey to several addictions (Drugs, alcohol, sex, pornography, gambling, etc.). Such addictions also make people incapable of making conscious decisions. Most of their decisions are made under the influence of their addiction.

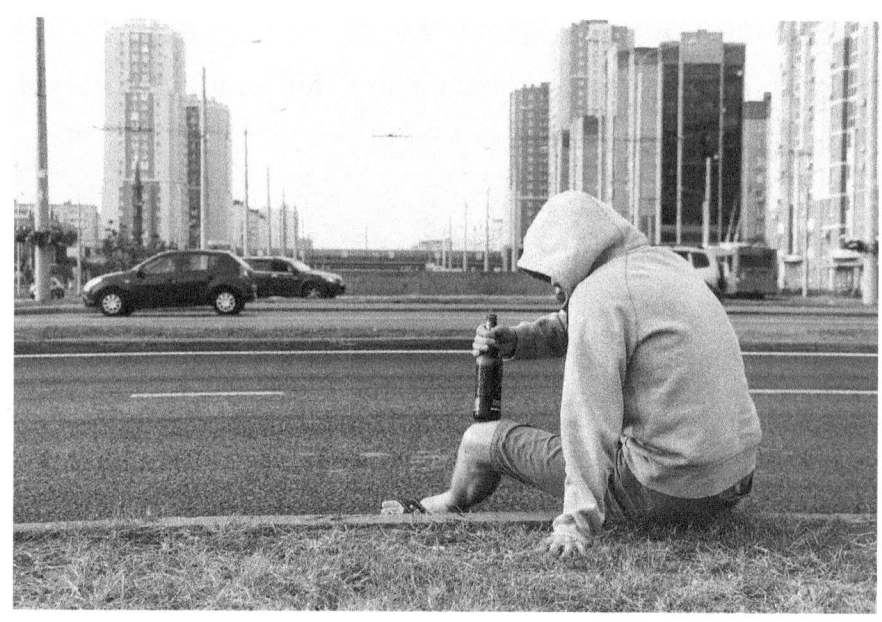

If a relationship is becoming unresponsive, abusive, tiring and painful, it is best to let it go. The longer you cling to it, the stronger impact it will have on your personality.

In such a scenario, leaving them is the best. You need to move on. You need to consider the fact that there is no chance of the revival of that relationship and neither is there any gain.

You Should Start Considering

The Possibilities of Living Without Such a Person

Living with people for some time makes them a part of your life. You start identifying with them. Growing apart is always a difficult process. However, you must weigh the odds. If the thought of living those people torments you, then parting ways is the best solution in the interest of both of the partners. There is nothing much left there to revive.

The Impact of Growing Apart

Ending a relationship however bad is tough. All relationships have their memories and bitter-sweet moments. You simply can't hold on to one aspect of the relationship and leave another. When you sever the ties, it must be complete. There will be some pain and discomfort as a part of the process. But, if you do not end all ties, you will be prolonging the agony.

Some people remain indecisive and try to do it slowly. They are never able to get over with such relationships. Their life and experiences always remain affected by toxic relationships. They are never able to experience true freedom or an obligation-free chance to move on in life. They remain stuck in the toxic relationship forever. If you ever want to successfully get out of some relationships, then cut-off all communication completely. This is the only way to free yourself and your ex-partner of all obligations. Get and give a new chance.

The Ways to Express Your Intent as Dispassionately as Possible

Ending a relationship can be a stressful decision. It comes with a heavy burden of accepting the failures and blames. However, the important thing is accepting the fact that the relationship hasn't been able to work irrespective of the efforts put into it. Try to be as dispassionate as possible in your decision. Do not go into fixing the blame or seeking responsibility mode. It will make moving on difficult for you. It can also invoke a negative, violent, or unexpected reaction from your partner.

The Ways to Handle the Possible Negative Reaction

Every action has a reaction. Similarly, your decision to move on from the relationship may not go down well with your ex-partner. There can be a physical, emotional or verbal outburst. You must prepare yourself for the situation in advance. If you know the person to be physically or verbally abusive, do this at a place where the chances of harm are the least. You can also do it over phone, email or messages. It may also not be that easy to move from a relationship for you emotionally. Some negative memories simply cling to you. Seek expert help and therapy. Do not ignore the need to get over with it for good.

The Ways to Process This Change in Life

There can be repercussions of breaking relationships. Emotional, physical or objective attachments make it difficult to move on. However, you'll need to learn to move. Moving on is a slow process that takes place with time. It is time that heals the wounds of tethered relationships. The best thing is to allow the required time to yourself to get over it completely. You also learn that moving away is a slow process. It takes place in stages. First, the longing goes, and then the attachments and finally, the memories fade away. Life takes its course on its own speed.

Hanging on to a toxic relationship can be a highly stressful process. It makes you anxious and unable to function normally. Your efficiency, performance, and focus go down. Therefore, if a relationship is making you feel suffocated, tormented, or abused, it is in your best interest to move out of it.

Having a positive attitude towards life is very important for recovering from such painful experiences.

A positive attitude gives you the power to move on and give your life a new start. Positive attitude in life enables you to live life enthusiastically and fully like a winner.

Chapter 10: The Magic of Positive Thinking

Positive thinking is a tool that can help you in easily navigating through the worst problems. It keeps you motivated and reduces the intensity of the problem. People believe that some problems are big while others are small. However, all problems are alike, they are simply problems. The problems you feel you can handle easily look small while the others look big. A problem that may look small to you may be an impossibility for others. It is simply a matter of perception. We are a sum total of all our fears. If we think we can manage something, we will, otherwise, we won't.

Positivity has a very strong impact on stress, anxiety, and worries. A positive mind looks at the problems to solve them. It doesn't let the problems take a toll. Positive people have the least amount of stress in their lives.

Decluttering your mind can help you in keeping you positive. It keeps your goals clear and takes away the confusions.

Some of the Ways to Clear the Clutter and Keeping Yourself Positive

Know What You Want

Clarity of desires is the first step towards having an uncluttered mind. Always have clarity about the things you want. This stops cropping up of unnecessary desires. You remain clear and focused.

Know Why You Want It

Not knowing the reason for having a particular desire leads to ambiguity. This gives way to a trend where you start wishing to have anything and everything. It makes you feel more and more miserable. The more you want, the less you can have and it leads to negativity. Always have a proper justification for the things that you desire and the role they are going to have in your happiness. This keeps your mind free from clutter and removes the reasons for stress.

Stay Positive

Always stay positive about achieving your goals. Pay undivided attention to your goals and remain focused. It will help you in staying positive.

Set Long-Term and Short-Term Goals

Your short-term and long-term goals in life should be clear. Plan your life. Having set goals helps you in forming a strategy to achieve it. You can set small milestones that give the feeling of accomplishments. Without these goals, there would never be a sense of accomplishment in life.

Set Priorities

Keep your priorities clear. Ambiguous priorities keep your judgment clouded. You feel distracted and keep hip-hopping between things. Lack of direction keeps your mind cluttered. You feel more stress and worried about your decisions. If you want to lead a positive life then keeping your priorities clear is very important.

Identify the Challenges

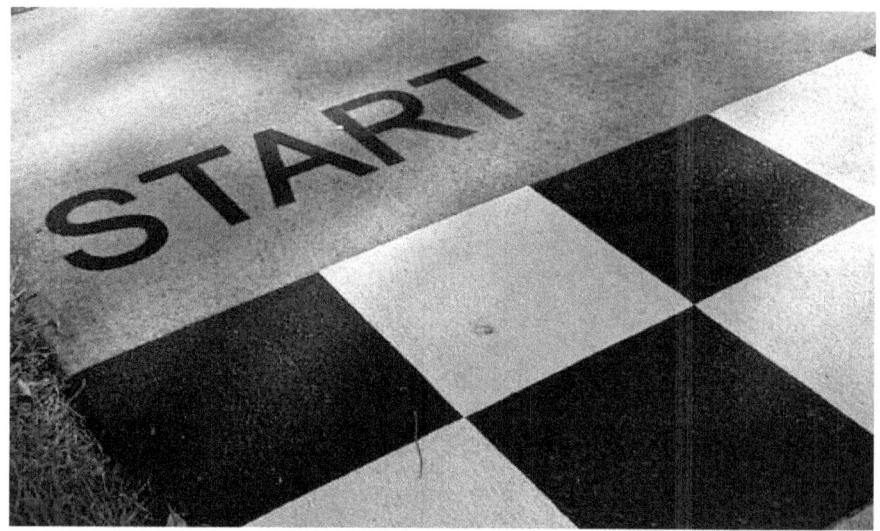

Know the challenges in front of you. Clear goals make the challenges clear. This eliminates the chances of surprises. You can plan properly in life and move in a focused manner. It is an important step towards a positive attitude in life reducing stress and clearing the mental clutter.

Write Your Thoughts on Paper

Whenever in doubt, write the problems on paper. Excessive rambling of thoughts in mind can cloud your judgment. It can make you feel apprehensive or indecisive. It also plants the seeds of negativity in mind. Therefore, whenever in doubt, write down the things troubling you on paper. This helps in analyzing the problems one at a time. You stay more focused and positive.

A positive attitude is a great gift. It makes your personality stand out in the crowd. A person with a positive attitude inspires others. A positive attitude can make even the bigger problems look small.

You are simply not born with a positive attitude but develop it by adopting some positive habits.

Some of the Rules to Develop the Magic of Positive Attitude

Be Optimistic

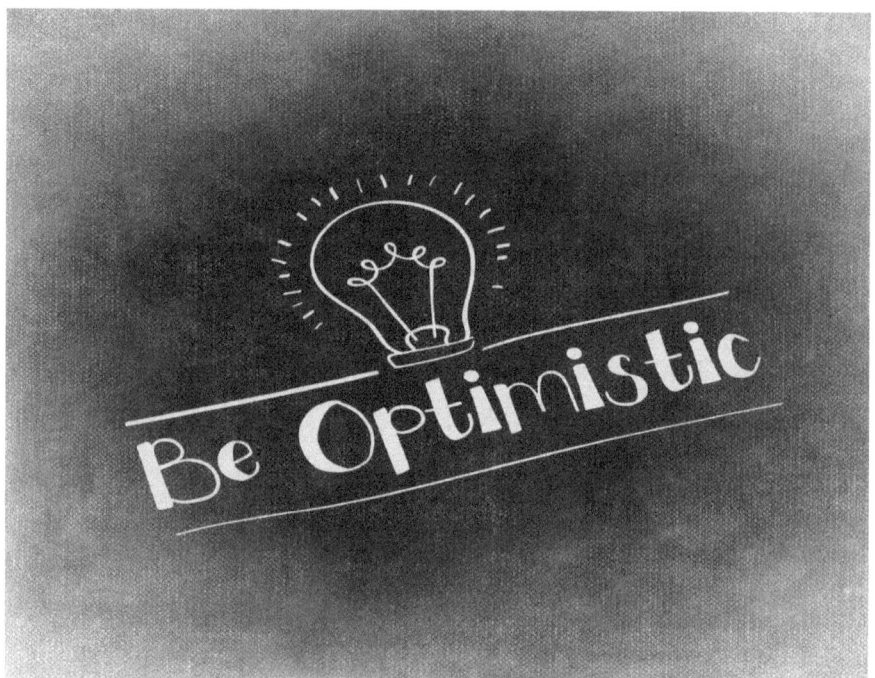

Optimism is the habit of having a positive outlook on things. An optimist person thinks more about the boons than banes. He/she is more inspired by the solution than troubled by the problem. The problem remains the same, only the way to see the problem changes and it makes all the difference in the world.

Be Grateful

Negativity is a reflection of your depressing attitude towards the world. You look at things negatively when you fail to notice the promise in things. Being grateful is a way to develop a positive attitude. When you are grateful about the things and people around, you are better able to utilize their potential.

Take Ownership of Your Life

A person with low self-esteem and negative outlook will never be able to take ownership of life or happiness. A regressive attitude keeps you burdened. You rely too much on others for providing happiness. You fail to look at the good things in life and in yourself. If you want to develop a positive attitude, then stop looking for happiness outside. Take ownership of your life and happiness and be more content and confident.

Remove Negative People from Your Life

Negative people can have a huge influence on life. They drag you down and cloud your judgment. Negativity has a strong impact on thinking patterns. If you are keeping a company of negative people that the chances are high that you'll soon start getting influenced by the way they think. They are discouraging and demoralizing. Negative people look at the problems with a very pessimistic view. They assume and would try to convince you to believe that problems at hand cannot be solved. Soon, your thinking patterns also start to change and you become less confident. Avoiding the company of such people is the best for a positive attitude.

Lead a Healthy Life

A healthy lifestyle is very important for being positive. An unwell body cannot remain beaming with confidence and positivity. If you want to remain positive, then adopting a healthy lifestyle is very important. This gives you a chance to keep yourself healthy and you become more appreciative of yourself.

Use Positive Affirmations as a Part of Life

Positive affirmations help in making you more confident and have a positive outlook. You must use positive affirmations daily to praise the things around you and look at the things from a positive perspective. This keeps you confident and motivated.

Be Patient

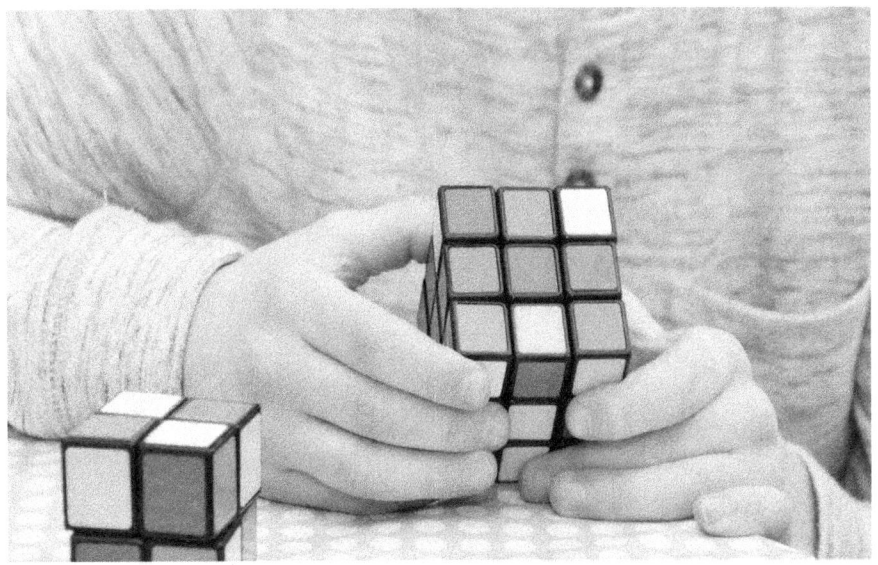

Patience is the key to problem-solving. Many things take their own course and can't be sped up. Impatience can make you feel anxious and stressed. Patience is the key to solving most of the problems in the world. A positive person is always patient about problems and remains focused on the solutions.

Chapter 11: 7 Steps Can Help You In Clearing Mental Clutter And Leading A Happy Life

These days life is prosperous and comfortable, but it isn't happy and stress-free. We are always struggling with ourselves and making desperate attempts to bring things in sync. Simplicity and peace are two natural things that have become non-existent.

Step 1: Let Go of the Baggage of the Past

The ghost of the past is tough to go. The harder we try to push it, the more resounding it gets. It comes to haunt at the most inconvenient times. It should come as no surprise that you always remember everything bad that has happened in your life. Your mind is a terrific storage device.

It has unlimited storage ability. Scientists believe that you can record more than 2.5 petabytes of data in your brain and still have space left for more. It actually translates to 300 million hours of video recording space. This is huge.

It means that all the things that have happened in your life, positive or negative, are recorded in your mind. However, your mind also has a strong response to negative things as it feels the need to keep playing them, again and again, to keep you safe from falling into the same kind of situation. It is a survival mechanism designed for good.

The problem begins when your mind starts playing the negative things obsessively and makes it impossible for you to start fresh. It makes wiping the slate clean tough. Your mind clutter has an important role to play in this. You let your past remain heavy on you. The solace of victimhood, the desperation to remain safe and vulnerability are some of the strong reasons. These feelings encroach your productive space. They leave no room for positive thinking.

This all happens because you are not being mindful. You have allowed your mind to remain cluttered by negative experiences and want to be in a safe sanctuary.

Let's consider a small story. Once there was a farmer. He had a big farm but he had bad luck in the past harvests. Sometimes the harvests got affected by droughts and sometimes pest attacks killed the harvest. The farmer decided he had had enough of this nonsense. He wouldn't bear this nonsense again as his harvests were getting ruined anyway. So, he decided to play it safe and planted nothing. Was that a solution? It was definitely not a solution. Earlier the farmer had a fear that his harvest would get affected by rain or pests. There was a possibility that he may not get the full harvest. But, his actions made it a certainty that he will not get anything at all. Playing safe is sometimes the worst move. The baggage of the past does this to you.

If you let your mind and thoughts rule your world then you will rot in a corner without ever seeing the light of the day. It will keep telling you that the world is full of dangers and risks.

Learning from the mistakes of the past and letting it go is the only way to excel in this world. If your mind is cluttered with worries it will never be able to learn and succeed. It will lack the required potential. A cluttered mind is never able to make the distinction between a safe decision and a fearful decision.

Safe decisions are based on reality. They have their basis on the possible consequences of decisions and they invoke remedial precautions. The farmer could have made alternative irrigation arrangements. He could have employed pest control measures. Even if he hadn't done any of these the probability of getting a harvest was 50-50. But, he took a fearful decision of doing nothing. The result was a guarantee of having nothing at all. Fearful decisions come from your insecurities and they keep getting stronger. If you do not learn to fight them, they will degrade you and make you sub-human with no capability to enjoy this life.

Don't Believe Everything You Think

Being a Phony Soothsayer - Do not Determine the Results in Advance

Fears of the past keep telling you that you have failed once. They cloud your thinking. If you start listening to that voice and relying on it without clarity, you will fall into a trap. Fear can be your worst enemy if it leads to inaction. The action carried out with fear in mind makes you cautious but inaction is deadly.

It is in our instincts to avoid danger as long as it is possible, but sometimes, waiting for too long is even more dangerous. You may think that you may fail in accomplishing something as you failed earlier but if you believe in it, you will fail for sure.

A cluttered mind has generally 4 kinds of baseless fears.

Fear to Fail

If you have failed at something, your mind will trigger nervousness whenever you get in a similar situation. Suppose you failed at one job interview. Your mind will make you nervous whenever you go for the next interview. It will keep telling that you'll fail as you had failed the previous time. Your mind is not thinking clearly. It is full of the past baggage of failure. You will have to clear your mind of such thoughts and remind yourself of your merits for the position.

Remind yourself that you came for the interview as you thought yourself capable for the job. You have the abilities and therefore, there is no reason to be so sure of failure even this time. Your failure in the previous interview can have several reasons. Even if it was your inability to answer some questions, the required thing to do is to work on that part and not to worry about the results. You must make your mind understand that only action is in your hand. The consequences of the actions are beyond your control and therefore they are none of your business. By not risking failure you are failing for sure. Decluttering your mind of such thoughts is the only way to overcome this fear.

The same happens in the case of failed relationships. People start considering failure in relationships of people as definite. It is not. Every individual and relationship is unique. It will have its own set of problems, but they will be unique.

Fear of Getting Rejected

Rejection is heavy. Most people can't take rejection well. Either it is on personal front or professional, people react to rejections in a very erratic manner. However, the baggage of getting rejected once never leaves the mind. When you find yourself in the same position, your instinct tells you to back off or you can face a similar fate. To an extent your mind is correct. There is a probability that you might get rejected even this time. But, it will have a learning curve as you will be able to understand the reasons for getting rejected clearly. Most people take a fearful decision and play it safe. They will never get accepted as they have surrendered to a lost fate. They will carry the baggage of getting rejected for the whole of their life and never get accepted ever.

You made a proposal in front of your boss and it was rejected once. There is nothing to get ridiculed by the rejection. Ponder over the merits of the proposal and prepare it in a better way in future.

You proposed to a girl and she rejected. She was not the only girl in the world. Maybe you didn't possess the qualities she was looking for. Maybe you approached in a wrong way. There can be hundreds of reasons for your proposal to get rejected. Not trying again with any other girl would mean not having any other girl in your life ever. It is even worse than getting rejected.

Your mind has the ability to play scenarios again and again. Use it to your own advantage. Recreate the scenario and learn the reasons for getting rejected. Do not carry the baggage for the whole of your life. If your mind remains cluttered and overloaded with the fear of getting rejected you will become a recipe for disaster.

Fear of Being Inadequate

This is a fear that most people harbor in their hearts to some extent. It begins with hesitation and leads to inaction. You may feel that you want to do something but you aren't good enough to do it. Your fear may be correct. But, this is why we as human beings have a gift of learning. Simply assuming that you are inadequate will keep you that way. If you feel incapable of doing something, then learn. It is as simple as that. Your mind has the ability to learn but a cluttered mind will always keep thinking about the things it isn't rather than focusing on what it can be. Brooding over some inadequacies will take you nowhere. This road ends right there. You are standing in a cul-de-sac. Knowledge is the ride you need.

Fear of Unworthiness

This is a fear that also comes with the baggage of past. When you keep failing or keep getting rejected, you start feeling yourself to be unworthy. It will crush you down and decimate you. Simply because you had some failures in the past doesn't make you any less human. Rome wasn't built in a day. The story of most successful people has been a story of continuous failures. But, they didn't end up considering themselves failures. Walt Disney was told that he had no creativity. Steve Jobs was thrown out of his own company. Abraham Lincoln lost nearly all elections before getting elected as the President of America. The people who succeed in their first attempt itself are called to have beginners luck, not success streak. Success needs to be perfected with patience. It cannot come from a person who considers himself or herself unworthy or doing something. The feeling of unworthiness is a diversion created by your mind to keep you safe from facing failures and rejections. But, it also keeps you away from success in life. If you are having thoughts of unworthiness in life then you need to wipe your slate clean. Figure out the reasons that prompt such feelings. Devise a way to get over the impediments and then triumph.

A cluttered mind will keep invoking these fears. It will keep your judgment shrouded. It will never let you see clearly. Its instincts are to keep you safe. It builds a safe sanctuary for you. However, it will take you nowhere. If you want to succeed in life and your relationships then you will have to declutter your mind. You will have to begin thinking rationally. Rational thinking doesn't mean you need to take unnecessary risks but it means taking calculated risks. When you take calculated risks, you know the amount of fall you can take and you are already prepared for that. You are prepared for it.

Life is about hoping for the best and being prepared for the worst. It is human nature to take risks. When you are born, you know no fear. You are fearless. You can put your hands in fire without fearing the consequence. But, once you get burnt you understand that fire isn't meant to play. But, this doesn't stop you from cooking food on fire for the whole of your life. You learn to harness the fire to your advantage. This is the beauty of the human mind. It can learn. But, to learn you need to be open to possibilities. You need to keep the baggage of the past aside and start thinking rationally.

We all have past that has good and bad memories. Unfortunately for most of us, the bad memories are the strongest. We never bank on the memories of our triumphs. We forget the good experiences in life and go in our cocoons of bad experiences.

A decluttered mind can enable you to bank on your positive experiences. It can help you in finding ways in adversities. It will show you the light when there is darkness all around.

If the baggage of your past is pinning you down and stopping you from moving forward then.

Make a Conscious Decision to 'Let It Go'

It is the most important step or overcoming your past. Your past memories will not go on their own. They'll keep weighing you down. The only way to succeed is to make a conscious decision to let them go.

- Write down the things that you feel are making you scared.

- Declutter the thoughts that keep making you feel scared.

- Write down the good things in your current positions and your strong points.

- Evaluate your current position and measure the chances of your failure.

- Take remedial steps to ensure the chances of failure are minimized.

- Consciously let those past memories go away as you have found a way to win this time.

Stop Playing the Victim Card

Victimhood is a safe sanctuary. You can easily place the blame of all your miseries on others and absolve yourself of all the responsibilities. However, it isn't a solution. Your position wouldn't change by assuming any such thing. All this is only happening in your mind. Even in your mind, you are a failure, only here someone else is responsible for the failure. In reality, you are responsible for the failure as you are not taking any action. The world absolutely doesn't care about what you think. It is a big brutal world out there which is judging others on their actions and not on their beliefs.

Declutter your mind and shun such cloaks of victimhood. Even if something bad was enforced upon you in the past it is gone now. Let bygones be bygones. Today is a new day with new possibilities. Face them as a new person. Consciously remind yourself that the world is not the same every day. The fate of your actions would also not be the same. If some injustice was done to you, it is a thing of the past. You may have been a victim in the past but you will emerge as a winner now.

Focus on the Present

Live in the moment. The people who keep reliving their past become a miserable history. They have no place in the present. You are still alive, but you are forsaking the right of being alive by living in the past. You are not a history book. You are a running chapter in the book of life and you should start behaving like one. Acknowledge the mistakes of your past and your role in them. But, do not leave living in the present.

Forgive the World and Yourself

When something wrong happens with us we start the blame game. We fix the scapegoats and malign them. It is our world of thoughts and no one has a control over it. You can keep believing in it forever. However, it is not going to help you even a bit. It will hurt and keep you pinned down. You will remain scared of venturing out as you fear the same fate again. You forget that if you do not go out again you will never get to know if you learned from the mistake or not or even if has the world changed. Constant blaming and complaining will impair your judgment of the world. It will also take away your confidence. Your trust will erode and you will remain incapable of doing anything.

Venture out in the world and forgive and forget the past. Start afresh with the new knowledge and face the world as it comes.

You can only do these things if you are able to let go off the baggage of past. It is a tough thing, but the most important thing to do nevertheless.

Declutter your mind and organize your thoughts. Overcome your fears and clear the impediments. This is the only right way to face the world and succeed. Do not fear the future as it is uncertain for everyone in this world. You are not immortal and hence you do not have the eternity to think about the past. Start living in the moment before you become a forgettable past for everyone else in this world.

Step 2: Eliminate Negativity from Life by Breaking Negative Thought Patterns

The power to think is what makes humankind superior to other species dwelling on this earth along with us. If you look closely, they do all the things similar to us. They are born, eat, grow, reproduce and die, just like us. There is effectively no difference between us and other species. The only thing that makes us different is our ability to think.

However, this boon easily turns into a bane when our brain starts indulging in negative thinking. If you feel that most of your thoughts are negative, depressing, and self-destructive, you are not alone. This is a malice that troubles most of the human race. But, negative thinking has deep roots in the survival mechanism of mankind and it has taken millions of years of careful evolution.

Humankind hasn't always been at an advantageous position in this world. We were weak and vulnerable. We had no protection from the climate. We were ill-equipped to arrange food and were practically defenseless against the beasts. Carelessness could have got us killed any minute.

To survive, our mind developed a negative thinking process in which it could play all the negative scenarios to devise a safe outcome. It is more of a protection mechanism.

If one person in the clan got killed by a beast the scenario wouldn't simply end there. Our mind would keep playing the scenario so that you can formulate a strategy to avoid such an outcome again. The mind played the same scenario; it invoked fear so that we didn't make the same mistake. It helped in our survival. This mechanism of having negative thoughts has protected us for thousands of years against all odds.

If today you are having a similar negative thought process going on in your mind, then it isn't baseless. It has its roots in the very same survival instinct that enabled you to survive even in the fiercest situations. However, there is a line beyond which anything becomes toxic. If you let your brain run loose without any control, then it will keep playing fearful scenarios to prevent you from taking action. Your mind knows that the safest bet to survive is to remain in the shell. The outside world is unpredictable and the forces are beyond control. However, becoming the slave of this mentality is dangerous.

Negative thought patterns arise in your mind as your natural response to certain situations. The extent of negative thoughts depends upon your threat perception.

Most of the times, there is no threat at all. You are simply scared to take an action and your mind starts showing you the worst possible consequences. This leads to inaction, procrastination, fear, and anxiety. If you fall into this trap, you are destined to fail. Inaction will take you nowhere. We have come a long way ahead of the vulnerable times. We are beyond the age of savages. This is a world that runs of dialogues, policies, and frameworks. There are calculated outcomes of actions. Even if all hell breaks loose, there is an extent of damage that can occur. If you do nothing, the damage is already done.

Excessive negative thought patterns forming in your brain are a part of mind clutter. Your mind is filled with too much negativity and it reflects the same in negative thinking. This can be a dangerous thing if it goes unchecked. It can make you indecisive, frightened, and weak. You will never be able to bring that winning edge in yourself. Your risk-taking abilities will end and you will become a fearful decision taker which means you will take no decisions at all. This is a pathetic state to be in the first place. You will lose all the control over your life. Your imagination and past scenarios will start deciding the way of your life. It will take a toll on your personal and professional life, health, family, relationships and career and more.

Become Conscious of Your Negative Thought Patterns

As said earlier, having negative thoughts is not a problem, but not being conscious of your negative thinking patterns is a big problem. Every person has negative thoughts. Only a toddler or a madman can be free from fear and negative thoughts. They are free from fear and it has no real meaning in their experience. You, as a sane person, have experience and hence, your mind will play negative thoughts about things, relationships, and events. The important thing is to remain conscious of the negative thoughts. If you keep ignoring the negative thoughts they'll become stronger. Even a small mistake will get played repeatedly and frighten you.

We all get negative thoughts either we are awake or sleeping. Your subconscious is always playing the scenario. Your job is to play the scenario with a conscious mind and rationalize. If you do that once in a day, you will be able to calm your subconscious. You would have quelled all the fears.

If you have negative thought patterns and the fright is overpowering you and clouding your judgment then start consciously analyzing your negative thoughts daily. Every day devote a fixed amount of time to ponder over the problematic situations at hand and the best possible way out. This will ease your negative thinking pattern and you will be able to work constructively.

Can't Undo Spilled Milk; Make Cheese Out of It

You can't remove negativity by negativity. If there is a problem, then brooding over it will not help. Think of the ways to overcome it.

On day to day basis, we come across several situations which have gone beyond our control. Crying over them will not help our cause. The only way to deal with such situations is to devise ways to nullify their effect. If you are late to work, then either choosing a fast transport could help or think of a better excuse. Brooding over getting late is not going to be of any help.

The same goes for negative thinking in real life. If you are having negative thoughts then in place of going deep into the repercussions, think about the ways you can deal with the situation. If a negative thought pattern has started and it is bringing in front all the bad things, start thinking of the good things you want and list the ones you can make happen. You can only kill negativity with positivity and you will have to make do with the things at hand. Try to make the best of it.

Stop Punishing Yourself

Negative thoughts are a torment. They lead to stress and anxiety. It is well known that stress and anxiety have a detrimental impact on your physiological as well as psychological health. They act as triggers that begin several negative processes. Your body starts releasing stress hormones thatlead to fat accumulation, lethargy, and heartburn, stiffness in muscles and the works. Your body reacts poorly to these triggers.

Trying to ignore these thoughts is going to make you even more anxious as your mind knows that you are avoiding them. You should adopt a 3-step approach to deal with such negative thoughts.

Vent: Give a vent to these thoughts. Do not be scared to think about them. Let them come out in clear. It will help you in clearly understanding the extent of the negative thoughts. Nevertheless, do not remain immersed in them. Simply ponder over them and get over with them.

Cap: Once you have acknowledged the full scale of the negative thoughts, it will be easier for you to understand their extent. They will be less scary. This is the time you can put an end to them. Devise plans to counter these negative thoughts.

Strategize: You have the scale of the problem; you have an understanding of it, now you simply need a strategy to overcome it. This is the stage where you can get help from several directions. Think of the ways to deal with the problem. You can take the help of your family and friends in dealing with the problem. You can look for solutions on the internet. You can read about the possible solutions. It will widen your perspective.

If you keep punishing yourself with the negative thoughts, they will keep intensifying. Do not do that to yourself. Deal with the problem in an organized manner. Clear the clutter of your mind and you will be able to think better.

Write Them Down

Writing down your negative thoughts is a good way to clear the clutter of your mind. If you keep playing the negative thoughts in your mind, they'll keep getting stronger. The same scenarios will keep getting repeated over and over again.

Write down the negative thoughts and get them off your mind. It will help you in sorting your mind. When one thing is less to mix, your mind is better capable of thinking. Nothing helps in de-cluttering the mind better than jotting down your thoughts on paper.

Consciously Embrace Positivity

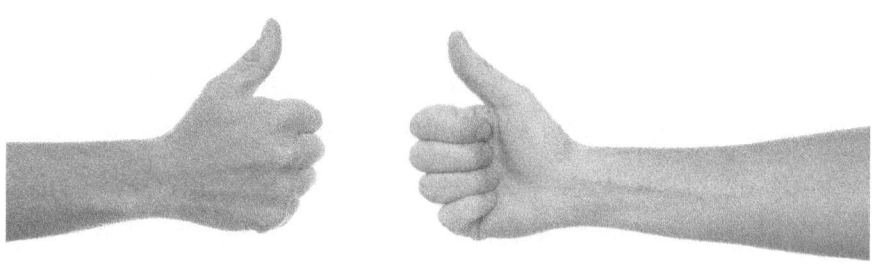

Negativity is a strong emotion. It gets expressed in a very visible manner and engulfs your thought process. The best way to deal with negativity is to embrace positivity. There may be a dozen negative things going around in your life at a particular moment but it doesn't mean the absence of positivity. You will need to remind yourself of the positive things happening around you. This will help in fighting your negative emotions. You should constantly remind yourself of the blessings in life. Think about the pleasant things in life to come. The things that you love or that infuse positivity. Take a break from the negative routine. Indulge yourself with some light moments. This will take off your brain from the negative thoughts. You will be able to break the negative thought patterns in an easy manner.

The negative thought process is very imposing. It has a very strong impact on your psyche. Simply trying to dodge this state will not help you. You will have to make conscious efforts to lighten up the moments. Positive things around you are very helpful in the process. Remove clutter around you. Organize your surroundings, as it also leads to negativity. Cherish your small accomplishments. These tiny steps to embrace positivity will help you in overcoming negative thought patterns.

Ponder Over the Merits of Negative Thought Patterns

Most of the times, negative thoughts are very imposing. They take off our mind from everything else. They instill fear. We are so frightened that we never pay attention to that extent. Fear has a gripping quality. It keeps us immersed. It has our unwavering attention. However, most of the times we are so engrossed in the fear that we overestimate its potential. If negative thought patterns are arising and fear is gripping you, evaluate its merit. Look closely if it can cause the amount of damage that you think.

Negative thoughts are there to caution you. There is no reason to become inactive. If you have a negative thought that makes you feel scared, then evaluate if it qualifies to put you in danger. Most of the times, the situation isn't that serious. You can easily overcome it. There is always a risk to reward ratio. Measure the risks and answer your fears. Do not take negative thought patterns on their face value. Think of the positive outcomes of your actions and compare if they are greater than the risks. You will have a better clarity of mind. Remaining lost in negative thoughts is not going to help your cause.

Stay Away from Negative Information Overload

We live in the age of 24 X 7 news channel age. Most of the times, the news is not positive as negativity sells fast and has great resonance. It is intriguing, and you feel like looking for more. This is the biggest reason, why most of the news items are negative. From social media platforms to the internet in general, negativity is widespread. The reason is simple, negative news has a greater impact than positive news. It creates curiosity that will lead to more TV time, more searches, more interest and ultimately more revenue. But eventually, you are at the receiving end of this negativity. It gives a bad start to your day. One negative news can shift your mind to the negative gear. You can start reflecting on all the things going wrong in your life and relate them to the news.

You live in an age where information access is instant. Do not begin your day with news. If you must, then look only for the news that concerns you.

Remain Mindful and Initiate Positive Action in Life

Learn New Things

Learning is a very positive process. It fills your mind with positivity and new energy. When you are learning new things, your mind is focused on possibilities rather than limitations. It provides a great stimulus to the brain. If negative thought patterns keep troubling you, then learning new things can give you great relief. They prove to be a great distraction from stress and anxiety. You get to use a greater part of your mind and it stops thinking about negative things.

Engage Yourself in Physical Activity

The extent of physical activities carried out by us has gone down considerably. We mostly live a sedentary lifestyle tied down to chairs or our couches. There is a lot of mental activity and stress but we don't get enough physical activity. This imbalance also creates a lot of negativity. Indulge yourself in physical activities. Gardening, exercise, repair or things, or building something new are some of the activities that will challenge your body. They will take off your mind from the negative thoughts. The nitric oxide released by muscles in case of intense physical activity also helps in relaxing your mind.

Creative Works

Creative pursuits like painting, drawing, playing some musical instruments are some of the activities that can help in distracting you from negative thoughts. They require you to exercise undivided attention. Your mind automatically drifts away from negative thoughts.

Deep Breathing Exercises

Breathing is a very basic function. We breathe every moment. But, we seldom pay attention to the importance of this crucial process. Missing our breath for a couple of minutes can mean the end of all. Yet, this important process never gets our attention. If negative thoughts are not leaving your trail then deep breathing exercises can help you.

Deep breathing not only helps in relaxing but it also fills you with positive energy. You get to inhale more air and exhale stress through deep breathing exercises. If you are stressed or feeling anxious, then deep breathing can be your savior. It doesn't need any preparation or arrangement. You simply need to inhale and exhale deeply. Focus on the process takes away your mind from negative thoughts and breaks the pattern.

Meditation

Meditation is an age-old tried and tested measure to ward off negative thoughts. It gives you an outside view of your mind. You get a chance to look at your thoughts objectively. It is a process of self-introspection and detaching yourself from your thoughts. It enables you to measure the thoughts on their merit. It brings peace and ends the inner turmoil. You can practice meditation for breaking negative thought patterns.

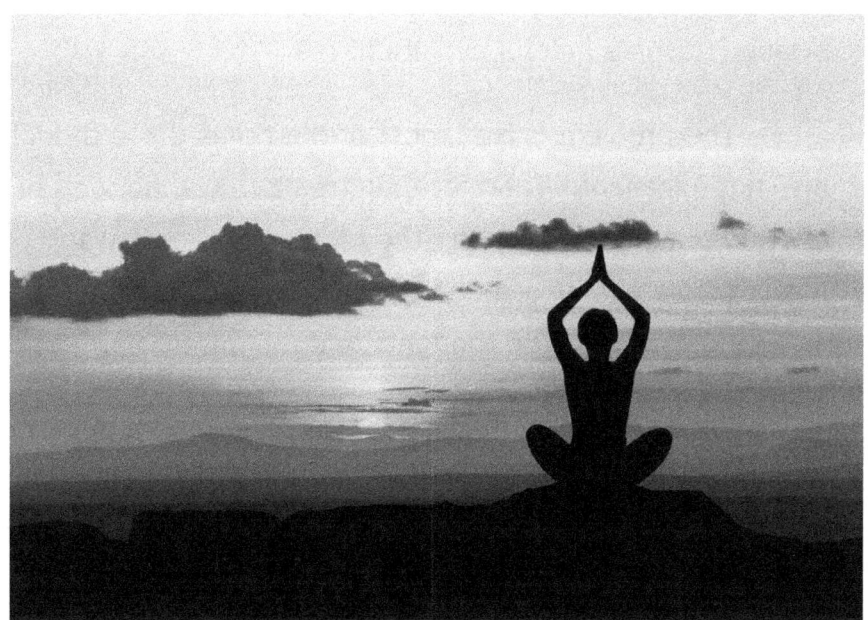

Step 3: Organize Your Mind - Control Unending Mind Chatter

Thoughtlessness is a state we all want to achieve. It is a state where our mind can rest without thoughts. However, the question is why we are so much against having thoughts. We have gained the ability to have thoughts after millions of years of evolution. Our mind has now got equipped with the power to think continuously. In fact, it can process a large number of thoughts simultaneously. It keeps thinking even when you are not awake. This is a helpful evolution.

The problem is that most of the times these thoughts are not pleasant. Therefore, in reality, we do not have anything against having thoughts, but we want the incessant rambling of negative thoughts to stop. We keep on trying to stop these thoughts and fail miserably.

The reason behind most of the continuous mind chatter is information overload. Your mind is continuously receiving information. Knowingly or unknowingly, you are grasping information from all quarters. News on television, movies, things happening on social media, things happening all around you and the likes keep filling you. You may never know but everything is getting registered. Your brain records everything and keeps processing them in the background. Out of this information, relevant information keeps popping in the front and your conscious mind processes this information. This creates a continuous chatter. This activity is beyond your control. It is very annoying and takes away all the peace.

It keeps you unfocused and preoccupied. Your mind remains cluttered and engaged. You face problems in grasping things quickly and show absentmindedness. This is an undesirable state.

Our mind has 25,000 to 50,000 thoughts in a day. Most of these thoughts leave a negative impact on your mind. This is the reason for most of the worries. A positive mind chatter may not cause any inconvenience. Famous scientists, philosophers, and thinkers always had something going around in their mind. However, they never complain of this mind chatter. The most obvious reason for that is the positive nature of their mind chatter. Normally, around 70% of the mind chatter is revolving around negativity. This takes away the peace of mind, increases insecurities, and kills productivity and efficiency.

Your mental chatter is a reflection of your thoughts. Your thoughts are a reflection of your actions and fear of consequences. Therefore, in reality, your mind chatter is effectively the sum of your fears and insecurities. A respite from these thoughts can help in relaxing your mind.

Sadly, there is no way to force stop your mind from thinking anything. It will start thinking more vigorously if you try to stop thinking something. Force of any kind doesn't work well with your mind. It is a highly equipped and efficient machine. Your thoughts are a reverberation of your actions. Mental chatter is not the cause of the problem but a consequence of your actions. You carried out some action or didn't do something and now your mind is pondering over the merits of your action or inaction. This mental chatter is never in present. Either it is about the past or future or both and beyond your control. You can never feel truly happy if your mind is always having this continuous mind chatter. It can have a negative impact on you.

Negative mind chatter will aggravate and agitate you. You will have no peace of mind. You'll feel more frustrated and tired. Mind chatter means that your mind is out of your control. You have no discretion over your thinking powers.

The best way to deal with negative mind chatter is to become conscious of the process. You will need to take off your mind from the train of thoughts and exercise better control.

Some of the Ways to Control Continuous Mind Chatter are:

Practice Mindfulness

Modern lifestyle is full of commotion. There is a continuous race to reach somewhere faster than anyone else but the goal is not clear. This creates a lot of confusion. People keep drawing their lines longer than the lines of others and the same pattern continues. In this race, our mind gets so occupied with the race that we stop living our lives consciously.

In the race to get a better living, we have forgotten to live at all. We are living unconsciously where most of our decisions are made instinctively. They are simply reflex actions having a tone of automation. This is the work of a cluttered mind. You remain so preoccupied with this race that you stop paying attention towards the pleasures of the journey.

Continuous mind chatter is a result of this immersion. It keeps you engrossed. It doesn't let you enjoy life. It keeps you devoid of the simple joys of life. The best way to stop this unending chatter is to start living consciously. The moment you become mindful of even your simple actions, this chatter would cease to exist. At the moment you are not paying attention to life. You are allowing this precious life to pass on silently. Mindful living helps you in experiencing life.

Life is full of beauty. Beauty in nature and in people both can have a soothing effect on minds. Mindfulness involves observing the simple acts in life closely. You start living in the present moment. Every sensory experience becomes important for you. You stop doing things absent-minded. It is a life full of observations. If you start living mindfully, you'll be able to feel the warmth of the sun on winter mornings. The sensation light breeze makes on your skin would become an experience for you. The joys and sorrows of people around will gain a whole new definition.

You become more observant. Your perception of things changes and you start experiencing life in new dimensions. If you become so observant of the present, continuous mind chatter will have no place in your mind. You would stop living in the horrors of the past or fears of the future.

Discuss or Write

Your mind keeps recording information and archiving them in your subconscious. However, some memories, fears, and incidents of the past never fade away. They keep repeating in your mind in form of mind chatter. The harder you try to push them away, the stronger and frantic they get. They take the form of unexpressed fears and if you do not give them a voice they'll keep eroding your peace. The best way to deal with this mind chatter is to give them an expression.

Talking to your friends and family is the best way to bring out these thoughts. Discussing them will help in understanding them in reality. They would become less fearsome and disturbing. When you discuss such things with someone, the thoughts also get a different perspective. You get a third person view and your mind can come to rest. Writing them down is also a good way to end the mind chatter. Writing down takes away that constant ramming of thought from your brain. Putting it down on paper helps in decluttering your mind. Your mind comes at ease. Incoherent thoughts also get a shape and you are able to understand them better.

Accept Your Fears

Bad memories have an uncanny way of emerging again and again in your mind. They take the form of scary mind chatter. They keep you frightened and insecure. This mind chatter is the hardest to deal with as it has roots in your fear. Most people suffering from bad past have these thoughts. They keep re-emerging in the form of nightmares or waking dreams. They keep pulling you down and make you feel drained. They take away your enterprise and make you feel already defeated without even beginning anything. They are a kind of safety mechanism going overboard. They are similar to a security software taking over the machine and completely shutting it down to keep it safe.

These fears become stronger if you try pushing them away. They have been a part of your past and have their roots in reality. You simply can't negate them as invalid. The only way to deal with such thoughts is to accept them.

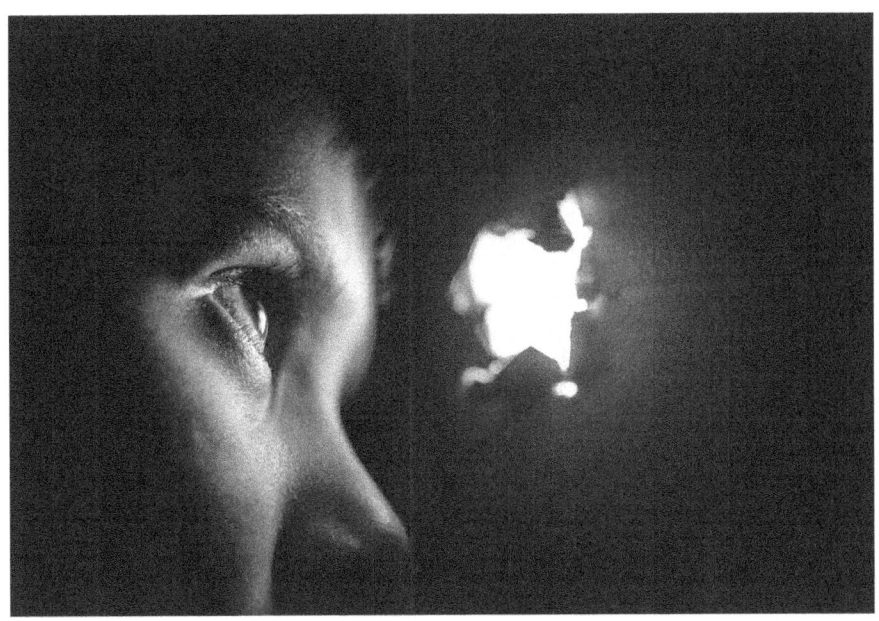

Accept that those memories are real. You must recognize that you suffered due to the past incidents. But, you must also establish that you have learned from them. You would react more rationally if the same thing happens again. Your approach to a similar situation will be different in the future as you have learned your lesson. Accepting such fears is the only way to get free from them. Accepting them will lower your threat perception and you will get stronger.

Step 4: Curate Your Desires with Minimalism

The expression 'desire is the cause of all miseries' is common. We all have heard it hundreds of time in our life. We have an unquenchable thirst. We want to have everything. When we are not able to have everything, we feel sorrow. This process is destined to fail. We can never have everything. We don't even have a definition of everything. Even if we get most of the things, there will be the lust to have more and it will lead to sorrow.

No other being in this world has such desires. The lion is the king of the forest. This beast has complete control over the terrain, but it also restricts itself to a perimeter. A full stomach is all that even the king of the forest desires. Its desires have boundaries. Only the human desires are boundless. An empty stomach is only among one of our problems. We are plagued by the sorrow produced by our unfulfilled desires.

Putting the blame of our miseries on our desires is wrong. Our desires are a form of energy. Without desire, we cannot survive. Everything we do is part of a desire. You get up in the morning because you desire. Achieving anything in life would be impossible without having a desire. But, leaving our desires unbound is the cause of the problem.

We are not conscious of our desires. We keep ourselves confused between the things that we need and the things that we want. There is no balance and it gives way to a lot of mental confusion. Your mind starts thinking that you need the things that you simply want. It starts a very negative process. One thing leads to another and you are in a big pool of confusion where you are simply unable to enjoy even the things that you needed and have. Unfulfilled desires create a mental clutter similar to physical clutter. They keep your vision clouded. You always remain in a pool of miseries. If you have a lot of unfulfilled desires then despite having more than most of the world, you will remain happy.

Happiness is not in having many material possessions but in the ability to enjoy whatever you have. Minimalism is the way to remain happy with your life.

We accumulate the unnecessary thoughts, information, and worries about things that bring no real joy to us. We keep pursuing dreams that may never have any real significance in our level of happiness. We keep trying to boost our inflated ego by wishing things and remain miserable. You may never know, but these thoughts, wishes, fancies, and dreams leave a very strong impact on your subconscious and your level of happiness and satisfaction.

The more unsatisfied, discontent, or wishful you remain, the higher will be your mental clutter. Your competition is not with the world. This life should be a peaceful journey. If you keep looking for happiness in material possessions, your life would remain difficult as this pursuit has no end.

The mental clutter created by unfulfilled desires is tough. It drains you and never lets you rest in peace. Unfulfilled desires even take away your chances of enjoying the things you possess.

Minimalism for Reducing Mental Clutter

Prioritize

The easy and simple way to remain happy is to determine the things that you really need in life. The priorities in life should be set straight in the first place. If your priorities are misplaced you will have the desires that know no bound. You will always remain unhappy and discontent.

You must have your priorities clear. You must set your goals in a mindful manner so that you can experience happiness. The people who set mindless goals can never be happy. They will remain unhappy even after reaching the zenith.

This is a materialistic world and aspiring for some material pleasures is not wrong. Most people would feel unhappy if they do not have the basic amenities in life. But, apart from the basic amenities, more material possessions can never give you happiness. For example, you need one home to live. There is no fun in being homeless. But, aspiring to have the biggest home in the world is a futile desire. It will lead to a race. It will be a race in which your chances of losing are the highest. Someone would someday aspire to have a bigger home and have it. This will leave you unhappy, despite having a very big home.

Having your ego satisfied should never be your desire. It is a road to unhappiness. It leads to a world which is lonely, sad and gloomy. If you want to be happy, you must have conscious desires. Unconscious expression of desires is dangerous.

Think clearly about the things that you really need in life. This will clear a lot of thoughts in your mind. A number of things that are on your 'must have' list may not be required at all. This will give you a lot of breathing space. Your mind will have more time to focus on the things that you really need. Either it is your career, relationships or goals, there must be clarity about their significance in your life and happiness.

Downsize Toxic Relationships

Relationships are very important in our lives. They give meaning to our existence. However, all relationships are not meant to last forever. For one reason or another people grow apart. Relationships do not remain cordial but your desires to be in them always remain the same. This desire is the cause of most of the troubles. A relationship which hasn't worked is not going to give you anything. If you harbor the desire to be in it, you'll be causing more pain and sorrow for yourself and the other person. Your mind would always remain occupied with planning to make things work. However, you must never forget that relationships are a two-way affair. The harder you'll try, the worse it'll get. There are some relationships that are completely dry. You simply aspire to have them. Such goals also drain your energy and keep your mind cluttered.

You must learn to get away from such relationships. Move-on and look for more fruitful and meaningful relationships in life. This will give you better clarity of thoughts and you will be able to channelize your energy in a productive way.

Rethink the Stress Price You are Paying

There is no doubt in the fact that day-to-day life has become very stressful. The work pressure, commitments, engagements, performance pressure, and deadlines keep your mind occupied. There is so much going on in a day, remaining mindful becomes extremely difficult. It increases the stress

and anxiety levels but you bear everything to achieve success. However, the real question is, do you really need that success? Most of us are running in a rat race which we haven't chosen. We are not running to win but we are running because everyone else is running. This is a mad and directionless race.

The race to excellence is taking a toll on your health, mental peace, and quality of life, but do you really want to be a part of it? Mindless pursuit of things is one of the biggest reasons for mental clutter. It takes away your mind from the real goal and you keep wandering aimlessly. If you are also feeling overstressed, overworked, and exhausted, then it is really high-time to think whether you really want that stress or not?

If you are not really driven by this race, then getting out of it is easy. If you are driving it, then reconsider the price you are ready to pay for it. Physical and mental stress from work and professional environment can drive people crazy. High-pressure situations, the demanding nature of your boss or clients, budget constraints, and several other similar factors can lead to high stress. It will increase the clutter in mind. Important thing is to consider the whole gain from this exercise. Money, luxury, or reputation can be the driving forces behind your pursuit, but in the end, they all boil down to happiness.

You must work on reducing the stress levels. Downsize the amount of work you want to take. Reevaluate the amount of gain required to keep you happy. This will help in decluttering your mind.

Most of the times, the things for which we are working very hard aren't serving any pressure at all.

Alexander the Great, who conquered most of the known world of his time, expressed in his last wish to be buried with open hands to demonstrate that you come and go empty-handed. It is not the wealth that you carry with yourself. This is the world where you experience the hell or heaven. You can keep collecting wealth for all your life to enjoy it in the end, but cannot be sure of the fact that you'll survive till the end to enjoy that wealth.

Desires will always keep your mind cluttered. They'll keep presenting new goals in front of you and shift the goal post a little further. Desire is like a carrot hanging with a stick in front of a donkey. No matter how far the donkey goes, the carrot would still remain a distant dream. It is a fruitless pursuit but it still keeps the donkey engaged. Do not let your mind deceive you into doing the same.

Step 5: Command Ownership of Your Happiness

All of us want to be happy, but most of us keep feeling miserable. Happiness is one thing that eludes even the most successful people. The people who look the most satisfied are sometimes the most unhappy people. However, the case is not any different for unsuccessful people. They also remain happy most of their lives.

The reason for unhappiness is discontent. We have given away our life and unhappiness to discontent. We are not in charge of our happiness. The things that trigger happiness are beyond control for most of us. This situation must change.

The 3 Main Reasons for Unhappiness

Discontent

We have formed a notion that we can only feel happy when we have a set of material possessions. The truth is that any amount of material possessions cannot keep you happy. In fact, if you look around yourself closely, you'll find that the people who had the most ended up letting go their possessions. It is proof that it wasn't enough for making them happy.

Our quest for material possessions keeps us feeling discontent and we remain unhappy. They keep the mind cluttered and we are never able to focus on real happiness. Happiness is not something that can come from outside. A child doesn't have any knowledge of possessions and can live happily. The day you learn to hoard you associate happiness with hoarding things and the chase begins. Do not let desires clutter your mind. It will make you incapable of finding happiness in the little things of life. If you really want to be happy, the first thing to do is to learn to be content.

Relationships

We all need healthy relationships. Healthy relationships fill the void in our lives. They make us feel content. However, if we keep looking for relationships to make us happy we'll keep feeling miserable. In that case, we become dependent on them. We give the charge of our happiness to the relationships. This is the beginning of the problems in the first place. Any relationship will only be fulfilling if you are there to contribute. The day you enter into a relationship to receive, you'll make it toxic. The joy and satisfaction of giving make the relationship happy.

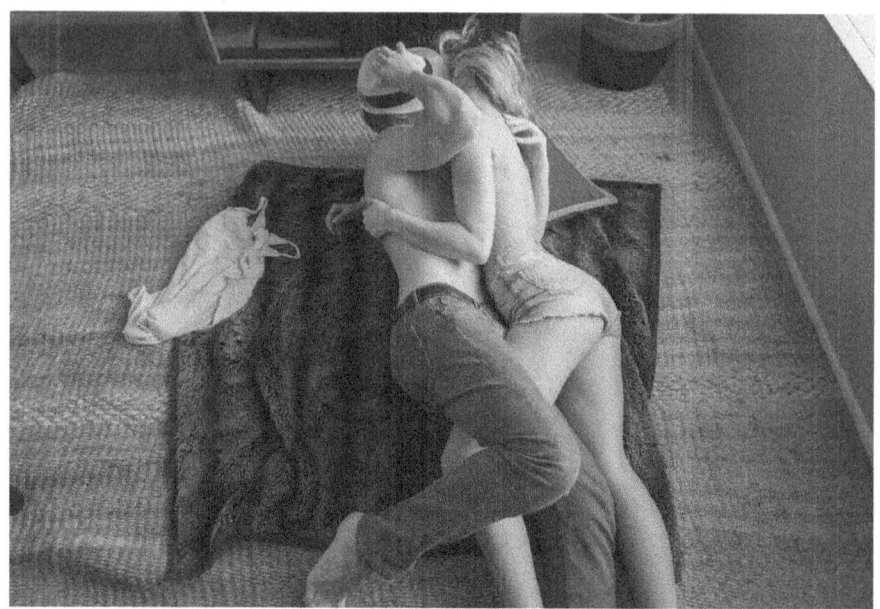

You cannot expect the relationships to make you happy. The relationships can only make you complete and unified. Happiness is something that can only come from you. Unfulfilled expectations in relationships clutter your rational thinking. Your mind becomes foggy and you become less giving and more demanding. This will kill your happiness.

Worldly Influence

We are emotional beings and therefore, we can easily get influenced by the outside world. However, overdependence on the outside world can take away all the happiness from our lives. The world is full of negativity and if you go looking for it, you'll strike gold.

The important thing is to avoid negative influence for remaining happy. Information overload, overdependence on social media, and unending quest for praise and appreciation are the factors that can kill happiness in your life. These things will kill the happiness inside you and make you gloomy.

These factors easily clutter your mind and render you incapable of finding happiness.

Take Charge of Your Happiness

Become Conscious of Your Mortality

We keep sulking about things. There is an endless pursuit of happiness and we constantly try to find it in one thing or the other. Think of all the moments of true happiness and joy that you experienced in the last 24 hours. Ideally, your counting wouldn't go more than half a dozen if you are very positive. Some people might not be able to recall even one incident of happiness in the past 24 hours. Now, think of your childhood. It was a time when you had to be made unhappy forcefully. Unhappiness required an outward force. Joy and happiness came naturally to you. You never needed outside stimuli to be happy. You are still the same person. The only thing that has changed is your perception. Now, you have more in your plate than you can chew. You have so many things on your mind that you are never able to rejoice the moments of happiness or experience true joy. Look at the other organisms. Their lives are full of uncertainty. They have no resources at their disposal. Their life expectancy is low. They have no way to entertain themselves, but they are calm and peaceful. They are not brooding like us or going on a pursuit of happiness.

We are so preoccupied with our search for happiness that we have started to look at it in the wrong places. We are the most fortunate species on earth but we have stopped counting the blessings.

Consider this simple fact:

Every day, around 200,000 people die on this earth. You are fortunate to be among the ones surviving the night. It is a blessing that you choose to overlook. You are not happy that you are alive and kicking. You are not an immortal. This means that you will die one day. Yet, you choose to ignore this wonderful gift of life so easily. Every day, 5 or 6 people close to the people who died will feel unhappy. If you are awake and all those people whom you love and treasure are also alive this is all the more reason for you to be happy.

We have become so preoccupied with ourselves that we have started taking this precious life for granted. We ignore all the precious blessings and keep searching for happiness outside. If happiness has to come, then it can only come from inside. You can only enjoy the tastiest food in the world in a true sense, only if you are happy. If you are happy, then even simple food will taste great. The same goes for everything else.

Do Not Rely on Others for Happiness

Happiness isn't something that can come from outside. If you are too much dependent on the appreciation of others to be happy, you'll always remain sad. The outside world will only acknowledge you when you are required. There are demand and supply equations in play. You cannot let your happiness be driven by the need of the world.

Find Your Passion

True joy only comes when you find something that makes you happy. Find your calling in things like traveling, creative pursuits, and hobbies that make you happy. Only the inner joy of accomplishing something can make you truly happy.

Decluttering your mind and finding the right happiness triggers is the way to remain happy. If you are blissful and happy in the inside the whole world would become a pleasant place for you.

Step 6: Cultivate Nourishing Relationships

Human beings are hardwired for personal connections. Our relationships complete us and fill the void. This is one reason we are always looking to form fruitful relationships. However, most of the times, the relationships we form become a burden. We are not able to sustain them or feel constrained in them. We start feeling the relationships to be a burden.

This inability to sustain relationships has become a widespread phenomenon in past some time. It is leading to unhappiness, discontent, and mental fatigue.

It is important to understand that relationships are two-way connections. Unrealistic expectations in relationships contribute to the problems. It isn't the other partner in the relationship that causes the friction, but your expectation from the partner. If you are expecting something from your partner, you may get disappointed. Even setting rules don't help in this case as it is not a matter of receiving but perception.

Expectations from any relationship cloud your thinking process. You come in the receiving mode. You start quantifying the unquantifiable. As a result, mutual trust and respect start fading. You become more and more demanding and less forgiving and accepting. Each and everything keeps getting registered in your mind and clutters it. The reactions arising in such cases are instinctive. They increase friction.

If you want to have healthy relationships, then being instinctive should be shunned. Mindfulness is the only way to cultivate nourishing relationships. You cannot let your mind clutter and prejudices rule your relationship. The clutter in your mind would make you unreceptive and unjustified. It will inflate your ego and make you unkind and uncompassionate.

Maintaining a relationship with another human being is a tightrope-walk. You are dealing with a being with the same level of intellect and completely different set of problems. You may be living in the same home, working the same type of jobs, and having the same friend circle, yet your worlds can be completely different. Every person has a unique perception of things. Individuals have their own way of quantifying problems. Every person has unique triggers of stress and joy. Measuring the other person with the same yardstick will create problems. The bigger problem is that if you have a cluttered mind, you will never be able to understand these things and cause friction.

The best way to cultivate nourishing relationships is to declutter your mind. Become more mindful and do not have prejudices.

Be More Inclusive

Mankind considers itself to be the most intelligent race on this earth. It has the power to understand and rationalize. It may be accurate to a great extent when it comes to understanding other organisms and systems, but it may work in understanding your partner.

Another human being is also as complex as you. Trying to understand the other person all the times is a strategy that will fail. You can never accurately predict the circumstances, outlook, and the reaction of the other person in a situation. The more you try to understand the person, the more alarm and defensiveness you'll cause. Relationships are not about accurately understanding but about being inclusive. You need to accept your partners with all the merits and demerits. It is the only way to disarm and let the guard go down. The harder you try to understand, the tougher the situation will get.

Listen

Most of the problems in a relationship simply need listening. When you are listening without judging, you are giving a vent to the problems of your partner. This helps you in accepting their problems and them a chance to open up. It increases the bond and releases stress. Your attentiveness is all that your partner seeks most of the time. Most people are capable of solving their problems and if they'll need, they'll ask for your help. You only need to pay attention to the things they need to get off their chest.

Mind Your Words

Opinions are double-edged swords in a relationship. If you are not mindful of the things you say, your relationship can go south. One of the biggest problems in sour relationships is speaking unmindfully. People do not pay attention to the things they say and do not foresee the extent of damage they can cause. Your opinions are only good for yourself. Do not push them on your partner or it can easily turn out to be worse than the prime-time TV debates. Mindful speaking is the only way to keep the guard of your partner down.

Don't Pick and Choose the Qualities

The main difference between human beings and robots is that every individual comes with a unique set of qualities. You can make any number of robots with identical qualities and features. We make like it or not, but this is the truth we need to accept. Nothing harms a relationship more than selective picking of qualities in a person. It raises their guard and makes them defensive and skeptical. Comparing of two individuals is inhuman. A person with a set of qualities also comes with a separate set of vices. If your mind is cluttered, you will not be able to see this. This selective viewing can endanger any relationship.

You must understand that relationships are not absolute. They can never be absolute. They will always be variables. It means that they will need mindful adjustments. They will need your careful attention. They will need your acceptance.

Decluttering your mind is very important for making yourself more receptive. It enables you to pay attention to things that are important.

Getting into relationships is fairly easy as attraction is the key here. Two individuals can come close due to the attraction. It is the point where only your strong points matter. You are displaying your strengths and pass on merit. However, maintaining a relationship is a completely different ball game altogether. You cannot pretend to be your best all the time. In fact, you cannot pretend anything at all. All your flaws will become apparent and the same goes for your partner. If you are not inclusive in your approach, then the relationship is bound to fall apart sooner than later.

To accept so many things in your partner and still be reasonably satisfied your mind must be receptive. A cluttered mind would fail you here. You will either end up pretending to accept or falter anyway. Both ways the things wouldn't end pleasantly for you.

Mindfulness, on the other hand, will ensure that you are in a ready state to accept the facts. You can take the facts as they are and live with them. This will ensure that your partner feels more welcomed and comfortable.

Therefore, decluttering your mind is an essential step towards building lasting relationships that can work for you.

These relationships will bring joy and happiness in your life. You wouldn't feel suffocated in these relationships and there will be no danger of them turning toxic.

Step 7: Develop Healthy Lifestyle Habits

Healthy habits that have a profound effect on your lifestyle can help in clearing the clutter a lot. Habits help in making good things a normal part of your life. They let you do things easily without putting much effort.

Clear the Clutter Around You

The clutter of any kind is bad. We keep accumulating stuff thinking that it will be of some use in the future. We all know that such a day never comes. That stuff only creates clutter and unnecessary obligations. Clearing the clutter always helps you in thinking better.

Keep your work areas and your home clean. The less mess you have around you, the clear your thoughts will remain. You will have better attention and your thoughts will not drift unnecessarily.

Eat Consciously

Food is a very important part of our lives. Whatever we eat, becomes a part of us. Our body is an accumulation of the food we eat. Try to eat as simple food as you can. Simple foods are easy to process for our body and have the least negative impact.

Keeping your food choices simple also helps in saving time and money. You spend less time on it and don't feel confused.

Eat on time and avoid eating very late at night. Healthy eating habits not only contribute to good health but also promote mental well-being.

Mindful Walks

The biggest reason for most of the mental clutter is the absence of personal time. Even if we are alone, we never give us the time to self-introspect. TV, internet, smartphones, video games, and other such distractions snatch that time away.

Make it a habit to go on long mindful walks daily preferably in gardens, parks or in natural surroundings.

These walks have a very soothing impact on your mind. You also get the time to ponder over the problems without distractions. You will feel much better. Mindful walks can be the best time in the day for you. You can use it for the very constructive purpose.

Be Mindful of Your Surrounding

Nature is healing. There is beauty spread all around you. Mind clutter takes away your ability to appreciate the beauty around you. It keeps you engaged and tired. You become oblivious of the good things around you and start feeling sad and depressed.

Becoming mindful of your surrounding can help you in becoming appreciate of things. You get a new perspective of life that helps you in solving the problems. This new attitude can also help you in pushing aside negativity in life. Practice mindfulness in daily life and make it a habit. Appreciating the little things around you will give you a very positive attitude.

Exercise

Exercise regularly. This is as simple and effective as any other measure. Make exercise a habit. The stress of daily life puts you under great pressure. Exercise can help you in relieving this stress daily and easily. This is one lifestyle change that can make a huge difference in your overall well-being. You will feel healthier and happier.

These healthy lifestyle habits can make your functioning easy and simple. They will bring positivity in life and help in decluttering the mind.

Conclusion

Thanks for making it through to the end of this book. Let's hope it was informative and able to provide you with all of the tools you need to achieve your goals whatever they may be.

Following these 7 simple steps can help you in clearing the mental clutter and leading a happy life. These days life is prosperous and comfortable, but it isn't happy and stress-free. We are always struggling with ourselves and making desperate attempts to bring things in sync. Simplicity and peace are two natural things that have become non-existent.

This book has drawn some main issues that steal your peace and make life miserable. It has also given a step-by-step way to resolve those problems. You can follow these steps and bring a positive change in your life.

Mental clutter is something that gets ignored most of the time. We all have it, but never pay attention to it. We attribute the stress in life to other problems. This misdiagnosis is a reason for pain. This book will help you in correctly identifying the problems in life and solving them in a correct way.

You can use these tips to lead a happier life and achieve success easily. It will help you in overcoming the burden of the past and moving forward. The past remains a big burden. It keeps you preoccupied, indecisive and stops from taking actions. This book will help you in dealing with the past positively.

You can use the steps given in this book to break negative thought patterns and think positively. It will help you in forming lasting relationships. You will be able to have a better approach towards relationships and have better satisfaction.

This book presents a comprehensive guide to remain happy. It helps you in taking ownership of your own happiness. It shows the ways in which you can end your physical and emotional dependencies for remaining happy. You can become the biggest reason for being happy.

I hope that you will be able to reap the benefits of this book and bring positive changes in your life.

Finally, if you found this book useful in any way, a review on Amazon is always appreciated!

Copyright 2019 by Andrew Copelan - All rights reserved.

The follow eBook is reproduced below with the goal of providing information that is as accurate and reliable as possible. Regardless, purchasing this eBook can be seen as consent to the fact that both the publisher and the author of this book are in no way experts on the topics discussed within and that any recommendations or suggestions that are made herein are for entertainment purposes only. Professionals should be consulted as needed prior to undertaking any of the action endorsed herein.

This declaration is deemed fair and valid by both the American Bar Association and the Committee of Publishers Association and is legally binding throughout the United States.

Furthermore, the transmission, duplication or reproduction of any of the following work including specific information will be considered an illegal act irrespective of if it is done electronically or in print. This extends to creating a secondary or tertiary copy of the work or a recorded copy and is only allowed

with an express written consent from the Publisher. All
additional right reserved.

The information in the following pages is broadly
considered to be a truthful and accurate account of
facts and as such any inattention, use or misuse of the
information in question by the reader will render any
resulting actions solely under their purview. There are
no scenarios in which the publisher or the original
author of this work can be in any fashion deemed
liable for any hardship or damages that may

Copyright 2019 by Andrew Copelan - All rights
reserved.

www.ingramcontent.com/pod-product-compliance
Lightning Source LLC
Chambersburg PA
CBHW070638220526
45466CB00001B/222